## DATE DUE

# Criminal Justice
## Recent Scholarship

Edited by
Marilyn McShane and Frank P. Williams III

A Series from LFB Scholarly

# Workplace Violence and Mental Illness

Kristine M. Empie

LFB Scholarly Publishing LLC
New York 2002

**Library of Congress Cataloging-in-Publication Data**

Empie, Kristine M.
  Workplace violence and mental illness / Kristine M. Empie.
      p. cm. -- (Criminal justice : recent scholarship)
Includes bibliographical references and index.
  ISBN 1-931202-50-8
  1. Mental health personnel--Violence against. 2. Dangerously
mentally ill. 3. Violence in the workplace. 4. Employees--Psychology.
5. Victims of crimes. I. Title. II. Criminal justice (LFB Scholarly
Publishing LLC)
  RC439.4 .E48 2002
  616.85'82--dc21

  2002010690

ISBN 1-931202-50-8

Printed on acid-free 250-year-life paper.

Manufactured in the United States of America.

# Dedication

Dedicated in loving memory to my nana, Dorothy Carleton, for her love, support, and friendship.

# Table of Contents

Introduction                                                          1

Chapter I—Routine Activities Theory                                   7
    Theoretical Elements                          8
    Empirical Research                           12
    Domain-Specific Victimization Models         18
    Property v. Personal Crime                   24
    Integrating Other Theories                   32
    Micro v. Macro-Level Explanations            34
    Summary                                      35

Chapter II—Violence in the Workplace                                 37
    Setting                                      38
    Environmental & Situational Factors          40
    Individual Traits                            40
    Role of Mental Illness                       41
    Evaluation of the Workplace
    Violence Literature                          48
    Summary                                      49
    The Present Study                            50

Chapter III—Research Methodology                                     53
    Research Design & Questions                  53
    Sampling Issues                              58
    Questionnaire                                63
    Pretesting Questionnaire & Use of
    Qualitative Methods                          65
    Administration of Survey                     66
    Human Subjects Issues                        67

Chapter IV—The Practitioner's Perspective                          69
        Defining Violence in the Workplace                         69
        Perceived Frequency of Violence                            71
        Perceptions Towards the Mentally Ill                       72
        Reporting Violence                                         75
        Precautionary Measures                                     77
        Summary                                                    80

Chapter V—Violence in Mental Health                                83
        Descriptive Statistics                                     83
        OLS & Logistic Regression
        Assumptions                                                90
        Multivariate Results                                       96
        Verbal Abuse                                               96
        Threats                                                   101
        Physical Acts                                             105
        Hypotheses                                                110
        Potential Offenders                                       110
        Guardianship                                              113
        Target Suitability                                        114
        Descriptive Findings                                      117
        Summary                                                   120

Chapter VI—Practical Implications                                 123
        Exposure to Potential Offenders                           123
        Guardianship                                              127
        Target Suitability                                        129
        Descriptive Data                                          133
        Practical Applications:  Where do we
        go from here?                                             136

References                                                        139

Index                                                             153

# Introduction

Since the 1980s, workplace violence has gained widespread attention (Laden & Schwartz, 2000; Southerland, Collins, & Scarborough, 1997). The issue of violence in the workplace came into the spotlight after a series of violent incidents occurred at postal facilities in the United States. One of the earlier cases involved a U.S. Postal worker named Patrick Sherill. Sherill killed fourteen people and wounded six others while on the job. This was followed by more violence by U.S. postal employees, resulting in 34 deaths and approximately 2,000 incidents of assault (including both verbal and physical attacks) (Southerland et al., 1997). The media attention given to these incidences resulted in workplace violence receiving national consideration and subsequently more research interest.

The National Institute of Occupational Safety and Health (NIOSH) released findings in the early 1990s that detailed the magnitude of the problem. Examining death certificates from 1980 to 1989, it was found that 7,600 employees were the victims of a workplace homicide (NIOSH, 1993b). Overall, homicide was the third leading cause of occupational death. National Crime Victimization Survey data from 1992-1996 estimated that over two million violent victimizations occur each year to persons while at work (Warchol, 1998). On average, 14.8 victimizations were experienced per 1000 employees. Some occupations, such as the mental health field, have had higher rates of victimizations occurring in the workplace. For example, in Warchol's (1998) study, mental health professionals experienced 79.5 victimizations per 1000 employees.

While workplace violence research has been given more attention over the last few years, there remains a need to understand how characteristics of specific jobs impact on the likelihood or frequency of victimization at work. According to Southerland et al. (1997), much of what is known about workplace violence is based upon two primary sources of data—the NIOSH study and the United States Bureau of Labor Statistics. As such, reliance on only two primary data sources leaves us with an incomplete picture at best. This is attributed to the fact that not all victimization is reported to outside agencies (e.g., the police), or is not reported at all.

Earlier research conducted by Block, Felson, and Block (1984), as well as the NIOSH research (1993a; 1993b), considered the relationship between victimization and particular occupations. More recent research conducted by Warchol (1998) also examined workplace violence across several occupations. Despite these recent efforts, there is still a need to focus on specific occupations, such as mental health.

The purpose of this study was to add to the current body of knowledge by gaining a better understanding of violence in the workplace. Specifically, this study examined the routine activities of employees who work in the field of mental health and the subsequent role that their routines may play in their victimization experiences. The research focused on a particular type of workplace violence, that is, violence committed by mentally ill clients against those who work in the field of mental health.

This particular group was chosen for a number of reasons. First, while available statistics have indicated that violence in the healthcare industry is a problem, especially for mental health professionals, information is limited because of reporting practices (Anderson & Stamper, 2001; McKoy & Smith, 2001; Peek-Asa, Schaffer, Kraus, & Howard, 1998; Terpin, 1995). Studies conducted using victimization surveys have shown that, while victimization is occurring, it is not necessarily being reported to the police, but rather to other officials (Peek-Asa et al., 1998; Warchol, 1998). This is important because studies based on official data, such as police reports, may lead to the underestimation of workplace violence in particular occupations. According to Warchol (1998), health professionals were found to report less than half of all nonfatal victimizations to the police. Thus, this study focused specifically on the field of mental health and obtained data directly from employees.

Second, there is a controversy in the literature with respect to the actual risk posed by the mentally ill (Appelbaum, Robbins, & Monahan, 2000; Baron & Neuman, 1996; Capozzoli & McVey, 1996;

Labig, 1995; Laden & Schwartz, 2000; Monahan & Arnold, 1996; Nigro & Waugh, 1996; Steinert, 2001; Warshaw & Messite, 1996). Some studies have suggested a positive correlation between mental illness and violence, and that the mentally ill are more prone to violence than the general population (Arseneault, Moffitt, Caspi, Taylor, & Silva, 2000; Eronen, Tiihonen, & Hakola, 1996; Hodgins, 1992; Hodgins, Mednick, Brennan, Schulsinger, & Engberg, 1996; Lindqvist & Allebeck, 1990; Link, Andrews, & Cullen, 1992; Link, Monahan, Stueve, & Cullen, 1999; Monahan, 1992; Rabkin, 1979; Shore, Filson, & Rae, 1990; Sosowsky, 1980; Swanson, Estroff, Swartz, Borum, Lachicotte, Zimmer, & Wagner, 1997; Swanson, Holzer, Ganju, & Jono, 1990; Swartz, Swanson, Hiday, Borum, Wagner, & Burns, 1998). On the other hand, some studies have questioned the connection between mental illness and violence (Monahan & Arnold, 1996; Steadman, Mulvey, Monahan, Robbins, Appelbaum, Grisso, Roth, & Silver, 1998). This study addressed the controversy through interviews that rely on the perspective of the mental health workers.

In addition, the current research also provided a further test of routine activities theory (Cohen & Felson, 1979), since it was used as the theoretical framework for this study. By gaining a better understanding of the routine activities of mental health professionals, it may be possible to determine the impact that those activities have on victimization. Routine activities theory is based on three concepts: motivated offenders, suitable targets, and guardianship. Cohen and Felson (1979) addressed changes in crime rates by examining changes in everyday life. Thus, the focus shifted away from the criminality of the offender per se to the behavior or "routine activities" of the victim. Shifts in activity will impact on the likelihood "that motivated offenders will converge in space and time with suitable targets in the absence of capable guardians, hence contributing to significant increases in the direct-contact predatory crime rates..." (Cohen & Felson, 1979, p. 593). A change in or lack of any of these elements may have an effect on criminal victimization patterns.

While there has been considerable research testing routine activities theory, the use of domain-specific models or constructs is less common; however, they have been used successfully in other venues (DeCoster, Estes & Mueller, 1999; Ehrhardt-Mustaine, 1999; Finch, 1998; Iyengar, 1989; Lichtenstein, Netemeyer, & Burch, 1995; Lincoln,

2000; Madriz, 1996; O'Loughlin, Flint, & Anselin, 1994; Wooldredge, 1998; Wooldredge, Cullen, & Latessa, 1992). Domain-specific refers to the specific places where and activities in which the victimization occurs. Domain-specific victimization models seek to increase explanatory power while maintaining generalizability by categorizing both life and victimization activities into domains that are defined by place and activity (i.e., work, school, home, and leisure) (Lynch, 1987). Also, domain-specific victimization models may help in determining the causal link between victimization and routine activities. For example, by specifically examining victimization that occurs in the workplace, differences between employed and unemployed individuals' activities may be discovered. "Classifying crime according to the victim's domain of activity at the time of the incident permits the exclusion of a large number of alternative explanations for relationships between particular routine activities and victimization" (Lynch, 1987, p. 285). By constructing a domain-specific model of victimization, routine activities theory can be more accurately tested by narrowing the scope of inquiry. This study specifically examined victimization that occurs in the workplace setting of mental health.

Furthermore, victimization studies that have examined the workplace have typically relied on household survey data (Wooldredge et al., 1992). While valuable, the data might be limited in that detailed measures of activity patterns occurring in the workplace are not provided. Appropriate measures of routine activities concepts must be employed in order to adequately explain victimization and increase explanatory power. To increase the explanatory power of routine activities theory, all three concepts should be included in empirical tests. Cohen and Felson's (1979) research has been criticized for assuming that offender motivation is essentially constant for all persons (Bryant & Miller, 1997; Massey, Krohn, & Bonati, 1989; Miethe, Stafford, & Long, 1987; Osgood, Wilson, O'Malley, Bachman, & Johnston, 1996; Schwartz & Pitts, 1995; Sutton, 1995). Furthermore, it has been argued that research studies have consistently put more effort into the conceptualization of target suitability and guardianship (Bryant & Miller, 1997). This study provided measures of all three concepts. Based on routine activities theory (Cohen & Felson, 1979), it was hypothesized that greater amounts of victimization among workers would occur when all three elements are present (motivated offenders, suitable targets, and lack of guardianship).

Considering what is already known about workplace violence, this study contributes to the literature by addressing areas that have not been fully researched. Specifically, this study gathered data directly from employees, both quantitatively and qualitatively. The data were collected from victimization surveys (as opposed to relying upon police or employer reports), as well as interviews. In addition, this study focused exclusively on the field of mental health and examined the day-to-day activities of mental health workers. The study provided a test of routine activities theory focusing on a specific domain—the workplace. The research also considered the risks posed by the mentally ill, as well as varying degrees of mental illness and the subsequent impact on risk of victimization. Finally, based on the findings, possible policy implications were suggested.

# CHAPTER I

# Routine Activities Theory

Many changes have occurred over the years concerning the activity patterns of the general population (Cohen & Felson, 1979). One of the major changes pertains to the amount of time spent away from home. Since World War II, there has been a shift in the routine activities of citizens within the United States. For example, there has been an increase in the number of routine activities occurring outside of the home, such as those associated with work. These changes affect victimization rates by expanding opportunities for potential offenders to come into contact with unprotected, suitable targets (Madriz, 1996). By spending an increased amount of time outside of the home—working, socializing, etc.—people may put themselves at greater risk of victimization.

According to Cohen and Cantor (1980), people who work in the labor market are at a greater risk of victimization than are those who stay at home. Increasing concern over the number of violent acts that occur in the workplace has brought this issue to the forefront and prompted researchers and others to address this problem (Laden & Schwartz, 2000; Lynch, 1987; Southerland, Collins, & Scarborough, 1997). While there is more than one theory of victimization (Cohen & Felson, 1979; Hindelang, Gottfredson, & Garofalo, 1978), Cohen and Felson's (1979) routine activities theory is the model used in the current research to examine violence in the workplace.

According to Southerland et al. (1997), "routine activities theory is relevant to workplace victims in that the whereabouts of the victims were known by the offenders and the victims were going about their normal duties when the acts of violence occurred" (p. 24). In addition, acts of violence in the workplace would qualify as an example of direct-contact predatory victimization, which the theory can potentially explain. Workplace violence also presents the three necessary elements of routine activities theory—motivated offenders, suitable targets, and a possible lack of guardianship.

## Theoretical Elements

Cohen and Felson's (1979) theory draws upon the previous work of Hindelang et al. (1978) and incorporates the earlier work of social ecologist Amos Hawley (1950). The model proposed by Hindelang et al. (1978) focused on the relationship between lifestyle and risk of victimization. Commonly referred to as lifestyle/exposure theory, it attempts to account for differences in risk of personal victimization as estimated through victimization surveys and other data. "Lifestyle refers to routine daily activities, both vocational activities (work, school, keeping house, etc.) and leisure activities" (Hindelang et al., 1978, p. 241). Hindelang and his colleagues found that victimization is not randomly distributed across time and space, but rather there are time periods and places that are considered to put a person more at risk. The model takes into account the demographic characteristics of the victim (age, sex, race, income, marital status, education, and occupation) and combines them with the constraints of role expectations and social structure (economic, familial, educational, and legal) to which individuals must conform. This leads to particular lifestyles in which persons will have both different exposure to and associations with others, including the criminal element, which potentially increases the risk of personal victimization. Thus, a person's lifestyle leads to different potential patterns of victimization.

Furthermore, if lifestyle differences are considered, it may be possible to both explain victimization experiences and to predict future victimization. For example, persons with certain demographic, social, and structural backgrounds may be more likely to be victimized because of the places which they frequent and the types of people with whom they come into contact. In addition, by making mindful decisions regarding the type of lifestyle chosen, one's chances of being victimized may be increased or decreased.

While there are many similarities between the lifestyle/exposure theory and routine activities theory (Maxfield, 1987; Messner & Tardiff, 1985), they are still significantly different (Tremblay & Tremblay, 1998). To begin, Cohen and Felson (1979) incorporated concepts from social ecology. Specifically, they drew upon the work of Hawley (1950) by incorporating the components of temporal organization.

> While criminologists traditionally have concentrated on the spatial analysis of crime rates within metropolitan communities, they seldom have considered the temporal interdependence of these acts. In his classic theory of human ecology, Amos Hawley (1950) treats the community not simply as a unit of territory but rather as an organization of symbiotic and commensalistic relationships as human activities are performed over both space and time. (Cohen & Felson, 1979, p. 589)

Hawley (1950) identified three temporal components—rhythm, tempo, and timing. Rhythm refers to the regular periodicity with which events happen. Tempo refers to the rate of recurrence or the number of events per unit of time. "Thus, rhythms differ with respect to their tempos" (Hawley, 1950, p. 289). Timing refers to duration and recurrence. "Rhythm, tempo, and timing, therefore, represent three different aspects in which the temporal factor may be analyzed, especially as it bears upon the collective life of organisms" (Hawley, 1950, p. 289). According to Cohen and Felson (1979), "these components of temporal organization, often neglected in criminological research, prove useful in analyzing how illegal tasks are performed—a utility which becomes more apparent after noting the spatio-temporal requirements of illegal activities" (p. 590).

Subsequently, Cohen and Felson (1979) addressed changes in crime rates by examining changes in everyday life routine activities. The focus was on the behavior or routine activities of the victim, rather than on the criminality of the offender. Theories such as routine activities do not focus on the acts of the offenders, but rather look at the lifestyles and activities of the victims in explaining crime (Miethe and Meier, 1990).

> [Routine activities is defined as] any recurrent and prevalent
> activities which provide for basic population and individual
> needs, whatever their biological or cultural origins...and
> include formalized work, as well as the provision of standard
> food, shelter, sexual outlet, leisure, social interaction, learning
> and childrearing...and may occur at home, in jobs away from
> home, and in other activities away from home. (Cohen &
> Felson, 1979, p. 593)

Since the World War II era, there has been a shift in routine
activities, resulting in more activities taking place outside of the home.
As such, the structuring of routine activities has had an effect on
criminal opportunity, thereby affecting trends in direct-contact
predatory violations. Predatory violations are defined as "illegal acts in
which someone definitely and intentionally takes or damages the
person or property of another" (Cohen & Felson, 1979, p. 589). Shifts
in activity impact on the likelihood that all three elements will be
present simultaneously—potential offenders and suitable targets will
come into contact without the necessary guardianship—thus, having a
positive impact on direct-contact predatory crime rates. A change in or
lack of any of these elements—motivated offenders, suitable targets,
and lack of capable guardians—may have an effect on overall criminal
victimization patterns. Thus, even if the number of motivated
offenders were to remain constant, a change in either one of the other
two variables may be all that is necessary to prevent or permit their
convergence in space and time.

Upon examination of crime rate trends in the United States from
1947 to 1974, Cohen and Felson (1979) hypothesized that "aggregate
official crime rate trends in the United States vary directly over time
with the dispersion of activities away from family and household" (p.
600). To test this hypothesis, a time-series analysis for the years 1947-
1974 was conducted. A household activity ratio was calculated from
current population survey data.

> From these data, we calculate annually (beginning in 1947) a
> household activity ratio by adding the number of married,
> husband-present female labor force participants...to the
> number of non-husband-wife households..., dividing this sum
> by the total number of households in the United States. This

calculation provides an estimate of the proportion of American households in year *t* expected to be most highly exposed to risk of personal and property victimization due to the dispersion of their activities away from family and household and/or their likelihood of owning extra sets of durables subject to high risk of attack. (Cohen & Felson, 1979, p. 600)

Ultimately, there should be a direct relationship between the household activity ratio and official index crime rates. In testing for this relationship, Cohen and Felson (1979) controlled for two variables—age and unemployment rates—that have been linked by other researchers to U.S. crime rate trends. Five crime rates were examined—murder, forcible rape, aggravated assault, robbery, and burglary. Larceny-theft was excluded due to a change in its definition in 1960. Auto theft was excluded due to problems in the analysis with multicollinearity. Of the five that were included, a crime was represented that is typically underreported (i.e., forcible rape) along with a crime that typically has high reporting rates (i.e., homicide). The other three are considered to have average reporting rates.

Cohen and Felson's (1979) analysis found a positive and statistically significant relationship between the household activity ratio and each of the five crime rate changes.

Whichever official crime rate is employed, this finding occurs—whether we take the first difference for each crime rate as exogenous or estimate the equation in autoregressive form (with the lagged dependent variable on the right-hand side of the equation); whether we include or exclude the unemployment variable; whether we convert them to natural log values; whether we employ the age structure variable as described or alter the ages examined (e.g., 14-24, 15-19, etc.). (Cohen & Felson, 1979, p. 602)

While a positive relationship was found, the authors were open to the fact that one of the risks with a time-series analysis is that the relationship may be spurious (Cohen & Felson, 1979). Hence, to minimize this risk, the authors ran the following tests to check for spurious relationships: Durbin and Watson, Durbin's h, the Griliches' criterion, and Cochrane and Orcutt's corrections. They concluded that the relationship was not spurious and that the relationship between the crime rates and the household activity variable held for both micro- and macro-level data.

As a result of this research, it appeared that routine activity patterns present an opportunity for crime to occur. In addition, the convergence in space and time of the three variables—motivated offenders, suitable targets, and guardianship—may aid in the understanding of crime rate trends. According to Cohen and Felson (1979), "the convergence in time and space of suitable targets and the absence of capable guardians can lead to large increases in crime rates without any increase or change in the structural conditions that motivate individuals to engage in crime" (p. 604). Hence, the absence of one of these variables may be adequate enough to deter a direct-contact predatory crime from occurring. While the research has primarily focused on two of the variables, suitable targets and guardianship, the other variable, motivated offenders, should not be ignored. In fact, they suggest for future research that routine activities be applied to the analysis of offenders and their inclinations.

## Empirical Research

Based on the theoretical and empirical work of Cohen and Felson (1979), a number of studies have been conducted utilizing routine activities theory. The theory has been used in the explanation of crime victimization that occurs in particular places and domains (Collins, Cox, & Langan, 1987; DeCoster et al., 1999; Ehrhardt-Mustaine & Tewksbury, 1997; Garofalo, Siegel, & Laub, 1987; George & Thomas, 2000; Lynch, 1987; Madriz, 1996; Maxfield, 1987; Norstrom, 2000; Stitt, Giacopassi, & Vandiver, 2000; Wooldredge, 1998; Wooldredge et al., 1992). It has also been used to explain various types of victimization, including both property and violent crime victimization (Bennett, 1991; Cohen & Cantor, 1980; Cohen, Cantor, & Kluegel, 1981; Ehrhardt-Mustaine, 1999; Felson & Cohen, 1980; Hindelang, 1976; Jensen & Brownfield, 1986; Kennedy & Baron, 1993; Kennedy & Forde, 1990; Kennedy & Silverman, 1990; Lasley, 1989; Lauritsen, Sampson, & Laub, 1991; Massey et al., 1989; McElrath & Chitwood, 1997; Messner & Blau, 1987; Messner & Tardiff, 1985; Miethe & Meier, 1990; Miethe et al., 1987; Miethe, Stafford, & Sloane, 1990;

Rodgers & Roberts, 1995; Rotton & Cohn, 2000; Rotton & Cohn, 2000a; Sampson & Lauritsen, 1990; Sampson & Wooldredge, 1987; Tewksbury & Ehrhardt-Mustaine, 2001). Attempts have also been made to integrate routine activities theory with other theories in order to increase explanatory power (Jensen & Brownfield, 1986; Kennedy & Baron, 1993; Kennedy & Forde, 1990; Lasley, 1989; Sampson & Wooldredge, 1987; Smith, Frazee, & Davison, 2000). Finally, the theory has been used on both a micro and macro level (Cao & Maume, 1993; Chamlin & Cochran, 1994; Felson & Cohen, 1980; Kennedy & Forde, 1990; Miethe et al., 1987; Parker & Toth, 1990; Rountree & Land, 1996; Rountree, Land, & Miethe, 1994; Sampson & Wooldredge, 1987; Schwartz & Pitts, 1995). Some of these studies have provided further empirical support for the theory, while others have not. Before examining each of the areas of research mentioned above, several general criticisms of routine activities theory have been noted and are discussed below.

Criticisms of routine activities theory have focused on the lack of available data for empirical testing (Kennedy & Baron, 1993; Sherman, Gartin, & Buerger, 1989), the construction of generalized models used to explain a wide range of facts (Ehrhardt-Mustaine & Tewksbury, 1997a; Lynch, 1987), employing methodological means lacking rigor and specificity (Ehrhardt-Mustaine & Tewksbury, 1997a), as well as using ambiguous, indirect, or inappropriate operationalization of key concepts (Cohen, Kluegel, & Land, 1981a; Ehrhardt-Mustaine & Tewksbury, 1997a; Lynch, 1987; Miethe & Meier, 1990; Wittebrood & Nieuwbeerta, 2000). In addition, it has been argued that routine activities theory is limited in scope and that it is only useful in explaining property crime (Bennett, 1991; Miethe & Meier, 1990). As suggested by Cohen and his colleagues,

> Much work is needed to establish the empirical adequacy of the theoretical framework...Further analysis of how routine activities relate to victimization patterns will depend upon more detailed data on the specific movements of people and property over space and time and the factors that increase or decrease their attractiveness as targets for criminal victimization. In addition, victimization data that allow for a more precise operationalization of the concepts employed in the routine activity perspective are essential in order to

conduct a rigorous test of this theoretical framework and to modify its structure where needed. (Cohen et al., 1981, p. 655)

In examining the literature, past research has primarily utilized victimization surveys and official crime data, as well as demographic variables (Kennedy & Baron, 1993). Sherman et al. (1989) argued that previous routine activities research has not used spatial data, but rather has relied on household and individual-level data. Also, previous empirical research testing routine activities has been limited "by the internal heterogeneity of crime classes and by the imprecise measurement of routine activity concepts" (Lynch, 1987, p. 283). Furthermore, the use of generalized models may not be adequate because criminal victimization encompasses a wide range of crimes, and it is doubtful that one activity model can explain all different types of crime. "Variables that correlate positively with one class of crime may be negatively related to another... and this can result in quantitative models with a low explanatory power" (Lynch, 1987, p. 284).

The same argument applies to the way that routine activities concepts are measured. The concepts—motivated offenders, suitable targets, and guardianship—encompass a broad range of diverse factors. "If these concepts can be more narrowly defined, then perhaps they might be more accurately measured in empirical tests of activity models" (Lynch, 1987, p. 284). However, while more precise models may increase the explanatory power, the generalizability of the findings might also be reduced.

Wittebrood and Nieuwbeerta (2000) have suggested that research include direct measures of risk factors—in the context of where a person works and lives—which correspond with one's daily activities. Also, they suggested the testing of more dynamic hypotheses that stem from routine activities.

As some scholars have argued, an individual's risk of victimization will be related not only to patterns of routine activities but also to changes in these patterns. Collins et al. (1987) and Lynch (1987), for example, argued that mobility on the job serves as an indicator of higher exposure and of lower guardianship, and will consequently lead to increases in the risk of victimization. A similar kind of reasoning can be advanced for changes in other routine activities. It is therefore worthwhile testing whether individuals who change their pattern of routine activities in a certain year have a higher risk of being victimized in that year than individuals who do not. (Wittebrood & Nieuwbeerta, 2000, p. 117)

For example, in a study conducted by Ehrhardt-Mustaine and Tewksbury (1998), detailed measures of activities and specific structural aspects of neighborhoods were utilized, which increased the explanatory power in the examination of victimization risk. The authors made the argument against using indirect measures. This has often been done in routine activities research due to the ready availability of such data. In addition, Miethe et al. (1987) noted that a major limitation to the theory is the lack of independent measures of lifestyles and the subsequent substitution of demographic variables.

It is near universally recognized among routine activities theorists that lifestyle activities are the most important variables to assess. Even so, however, scholars have almost always relied on status variables to serve as proxies for lifestyle patterns of behavior. Such inferences introduce conceptual leaps for the demographic characteristics of survey respondents to assumptions regarding such types of persons' activities. This reliance on proxy indicators raises serious questions of construct validity and has not gone unnoticed. Some researchers have suggested or attempted to reduce their reliance on such variables. However, the majority of research testing routine activity theory continues to utilize status variables as proxies for measures of critical theoretical concepts. One of the clearest instances of this is the use of marital status as a proxy for lifestyle. Most studies incorporating the use of marital status find that those persons who are married have a lower risk of victimization. The inferred explanation for this relationship is that married people are more likely to engage in home-based entertainment and leisure activities, while nonmarried people are more likely to leave the home for entertainment/leisure activities. The validity of this inference is less important than the fact that theories cannot be assessed accurately through the use of inferences. Theories must be tested using direct measures. (Ehrhardt-Mustaine and Tewksbury, 1997a, p. 185)

Furthermore, it has been argued that place should also be considered. As suggested by Felson's (1987, 1996) recent work, Roncek and Maier's (1991) research provided support for the importance of facilities and places. Specifically, Roncek and Maier (1991) examined the relationship between bars, taverns, and cocktail lounges located in residential city blocks and the corresponding crime rates for those areas. Prior to Felson's (1987) effort, reference was made to the crime setting, but it was never considered a central component of Cohen and Felson's (1979) theory. "Routine activities theory consistently discusses individuals' activities and the ways in which they put themselves at risk, but it pays little attention to the actual locales in which individuals become victims" (Roncek & Maier, 1991, p. 750). Roncek and Maier (1991) found that there was a positive relationship between liquor establishments and higher crime rates. Furthermore, the authors found higher crime rates among residential blocks with physical characteristics that allow for less guardianship and more anonymity. Sherman et al. (1989) also concur that not examining ecological data from the places where crimes occur is a major limitation in the research.

To increase the explanatory power of routine activities, all three concepts should be included in empirical tests. For example, Cohen and Felson (1979) virtually ignored the issue of offender motivation in their research by making the assumption that it was a constant motivation for all persons (Bryant & Miller, 1997; Massey et al., 1989; Miethe et al., 1987; Osgood et al., 1996; Schwartz & Pitts, 1995; Sutton, 1995). Massey et al. (1989) contend that the concepts and their empirical indicators have not been defined thoroughly. Of the three, the concept of motivated offenders is the most ambiguous. Furthermore, they argue, "obviously, one cannot predict predatory crime without positing the existence of criminals. But should the motivation, potentiality, or proximity of offenders be treated as an important variable?" (Massey et al., 1989, p. 383). While Cohen and Felson (1979) treat this concept as a given, there are pragmatic concerns and empirical problems that emerge. Massey et al. (1989) suggest that the concept of potential offenders be substituted for motivated offenders, as it may be objectively and subjectively measured.

On the objective side, each respondent in a victimization survey lives within a definable census unit for which there is a reported crime rate. The crime rate can be treated as a contextual characteristic that provides evidence of variability in the presence of offenders. A lag between the reported crime rate for specific offenses and self-reported victimization would eliminate any lack of independence between the crime rate and the incidence of individual victimization. On the subjective side, the presence of potential criminal offenders can be approached through the impressions of potential or actual crime victims. Implicit within the routine activities approach is the notion that people realize that criminal victimization is not a random process. This assumes that potential offenders pursue a rational thought process regarding target selection and that, conversely, potential victims make conscious efforts to reduce their risk of victimization. It follows then that potential victims' experiences with, or perception of, the presence of criminals within their midst are relevant (Lynch 1987). Perceptions of the presence of indigenous deviants within the neighborhood or community, perceptions of the amount and type of crime in the neighborhood, and experience with the actual deviant or criminal acts they have witnessed form peoples' sense of the size and motivation of the pool of actual or potential criminals who pose a threat to their well-being. These indicators, though unrelated to the criminal motivation of actual or potential offenders, do revitalize the role of the offender within a theory of victimization. (Massey et al., 1989, p. 384)

It appears then, that both the crime rate and a person's actual or perceived victimization experiences are important indicators in measuring the concept of motivated offenders. Until the concept of motivated offenders is addressed more thoroughly, its ability to account for differences in crime rates remains unknown (Bryant & Miller, 1997).

While it has been argued that more effort has been put into the conceptualization of target suitability and guardianship (Bryant & Miller, 1997), some have argued that more attention needs to be directed toward those elements as well (Miethe et al., 1987).

> Greater theoretical attention needs to be devoted to the relative weight and importance of the three major components of routine activity/lifestyle theories (target suitability, capable guardianship, motivated offenders). As our results indicate, persons who may be more suitable as targets and generally lack guardianship are not necessarily those who are more likely to be victimized by property or violent crimes. For instance, based on target suitability alone, some demographic groups should be at high risk because they are more physically visible and accessible due to greater activity outside the home (males, unmarried or young persons) or are more valuable as targets (e.g., older and high-income persons who have more valuable property). Yet, some of these groups (e.g. males, young persons) would be less suitable targets even if they were more visible and frequented riskier places because of their presumed greater physical ability to resist an attack and serve as their own guardians. (Miethe et al., 1987, p. 193)

Massey et al. (1989) also contend that the concepts of suitable targets and guardianship are not clearly defined. In their study of property victimization, they argue for more clearly defined indicators in order to measure these constructs. Specifically, there should be less reliance on social demographic variables as proxy indicators of the concepts.

## Domain-Specific Victimization Models

It may not simply be that greater theoretical attention per se needs to be spent on the variables, but rather a closer examination of the specific context in which they are studied may also be required. In order to increase explanatory power while maintaining generalizability, domain-specific victimization models have been introduced (Lynch, 1987). By constructing a domain-specific model of victimization, routine activities theory can be more accurately tested by narrowing the scope of inquiry. "This approach divides both victimization and life activities into domains that are defined by place and activity—work, school, home, and leisure (out of the home)—which may produce more internally homogeneous crime classes that can increase the explanatory power of routine activity models" (Lynch, 1987, p. 285). The rationale is that crimes occurring in each of the four domains will have similar characteristics. For example, it may be simpler to construct a victimization model at work than to construct a model of a specific crime (e.g., assault), and this process may maximize explanatory power and precision of measurement. Also, by focusing on a specific domain, it facilitates the process of discovering information on activities that affect victimization in that particular domain. As more information is obtained about a particular domain, it is more likely that better measures of routine activities theory can be constructed. With better measures, it is expected that the power of the explanatory models should also increase.

In addition, domain-specific victimization models also aid in determining the causal link between victimization and routine activities. For example, if victimization in the workplace were specifically studied, then differences between employed and unemployed individuals' activities may be examined more closely (Lynch, 1987). In other words, by looking at the crime from the perspective of the domain in which the crime occurred, it allows for other alternative explanations to be excluded. Thus, to increase the explanatory power and maintain generalizability, routine activities theory should be tested within specific domains.

Studies have been conducted that utilize routine activities and domain-specific analyses for home, school, work, and leisure (Collins et al., 1987; DeCoster et al., 1999; Ehrhardt-Mustaine & Tewksbury, 1997; Garofalo, Siegel & Laub, 1987; George & Thomas, 2000; Lynch, 1987; Madriz, 1996; Maxfield, 1987; Norstrom, 2000; Stitt, Giacopassi, & Vandiver, 2000; Wooldredge, 1998; Wooldredge et al., 1992). While utilizing domain-specific models in routine activities research has gained in popularity, there is still a need to focus on the work domain. In addition, current victimization studies examining work have typically relied on household survey data, which, while valuable, is limited in that it does not provide detailed measures of activity patterns while in the workplace (Wooldredge et al., 1992).

Appropriate measures of routine activities concepts must be employed in order to adequately explain victimization and increase explanatory power. Furthermore, "the behaviors examined in domain-specific studies are more convergent in time and space, so inferences to causal relationships between specific activities and victimization risk are more valid" (Wooldredge, 1998, p. 480).

In a study conducted by Lynch (1987), support was found for routine activities theory utilizing the 1982 Victim Risk Supplement to the National Crime Survey. The data included in the survey provided the necessary information to construct domain-specific victimization models and appropriate definitions of domain-specific crime classes. Also, the data were collected so that the analysis could be restricted to reported incidents occurring exclusively at work. Thus, the spurious effects of routine activities that correlated to work activities, but were not actually work activities, could be eliminated.

The supplement also provided data to measure four key concepts—exposure, proximity to offenders, guardianship, and attractiveness—which were defined and measured as follows. Exposure was "the visibility of or physical access to victims by potential offenders" (Lynch, 1987, p. 287). Asking questions regarding the number of persons interacted with in an average workweek and whether or not the public has access to the workplace operationalized exposure. Guardianship was "the presence of persons or devices that can prevent or inhibit victimization" (Lynch, 1987, p. 287). It was operationalized as the amount of local travel on the job and the amount of trips taken overnight. Perceived dangerousness was characterized as the "proximity to dense pools of offenders" (Lynch, 1987, p. 288) and was operationalized by asking participants about their perceptions of safety while working. Attractiveness was "attractiveness as a crime target" (Lynch, 1987, p. 288). It was operationalized as to how often money was handled by employees.

Of the four conceptual areas, perceived dangerousness had the greatest effect on the risk of victimization while working, although the other three were also statistically significant. Attractiveness exerted more of an influence than exposure and guardianship, which were similar in effect. However, it should be noted that the effects of certain variables were multiplicative as opposed to additive. For example, the effects of the exposure and attractiveness variables on risk were much higher when combined than might be expected.

In addition, demographic characteristics—age, race, and sex—were also used to predict risk of victimization. Lynch (1987) found that "activities performed as part of the occupational role affect the risk of victimization at work to a much greater degree than demographic characteristics of workers" (p. 283). Of the three, age had the greatest impact on risk, but it was weakly correlated to victimization at best. In other studies, age, race, and sex have been found to have a strong effect on risk of victimization (Cohen et al., 1981; Cohen et al., 1981a; Cohen & Cantor, 1980). However, these studies were not limited to the work domain.

Similar studies conducted utilizing work-domain-specific analyses have shown further support for routine activities theory (Collins et al., 1987; Ehrhardt-Mustaine & Tewksbury, 1997; Madriz, 1996). Madriz (1996) also used data from the 1984 Victim Risk Supplement and concurred with Lynch's (1987) research using domain-specific analyses. The findings also indicated that routine activities variables are a stronger predictor of risk in the workplace than demographic variables, when domain-specific models are used.

Another study by Collins et al. (1987) also looked at particular job activities to determine their relationship to victimization. Telephone interviews of 5,542 residents in an urban area were conducted regarding violent and property victimization. Only those respondents who were employed during the victimization experience were included in the final analyses, producing a sample size of 3,867. The variables included job activities (routine activities), household residence, marital and educational status, sex, race, and age. Violent and property victimization were measured separately as dichotomous dependent variables. Job activities were found to be a stronger predictor in violent victimization as opposed to property victimization. Some support was shown for the demographic variables—household residence, education, sex, and age. Consistent with Lynch's (1987) study, demographic factors were found to be significant on violent victimization when occurring outside of the workplace.

Ehrhardt-Mustaine and Tewksbury (1997) conducted a study using 1983 data from the National Crime Survey's Victim Risk Supplement. Like Lynch's (1987) study, they also examined the specific domain of the workplace and developed measures relevant to that domain. However, they extended their research by also looking at specific subpopulations. In this case, they looked at victimization differences between employed males and employed females. Survey data were collected for 5,647 females and 5,489 males.

The findings indicated that while routine activities theory provided some support for general work-domain-specific analyses, it was also necessary to include a consideration of factors that might have a varying influence on female and male victimization at work. In fact, they found that the sources of victimization for females and males in the workplace are different. Risk factors associated with female victimization included educational status and time of day worked. The findings indicated that women were more likely to be victimized if they were highly educated and if they worked evening hours. Risk factors associated with male victimization included place of residence, presence of security, and holding a job in the security occupation. According to the findings, men were more likely to be victimized if they resided in a metropolitan area, worked in an unsecured, open environment, and if their job duties included the protection of people and/or property.

In another study, DeCoster et al. (1999) also examined gender differences. Specifically, they examined routine activities and sexual harassment in the workplace. Sexual harassment is typically more common among females than males. In this study, gender differences played a distinct role in particular types of victimization, thus providing support for a distinction between male and female-dominated victimization.

Wooldredge et al. (1992) chose to examine a particular occupation as opposed to studying a number of different workplaces.

> Studies of work in general are more likely to generate results with greater external validity than are studies focusing on particular types of work. Research on single occupational domains, however, is likely to be more rigorous than general work-studies because such research makes it possible to develop very specific measures of work-related activities. Also, because tests of more rigorous and better-specified models may uncover relationships that are masked in more general models, such tests may be particularly useful for advancing theory. (Wooldredge et al., 1992, p. 327)

As such, their hypotheses reflected the work patterns of faculty. They hypothesized that personal and property victimization would increase for those who were on campus more often on nights and weekends, were alone on campus, had larger classes, mingled with students outside of class, and did not take much time off from the job. These hypotheses focused on the amount or degree of exposure a faculty member would have while working. Wooldredge et al. (1992) also hypothesized that victimization would be higher for those who taught in a building where their office was not located, who worked in buildings without security, and whose offices were located farther away from other occupied offices. These hypotheses centered on the amount of guardianship one would have while working. Also, they hypothesized that property crime would be higher for those who worked in departments that were considered to be attractive to potential offenders (i.e., departments with more capital resources located in the newest buildings), thus examining target attractiveness. Additionally, personal victimization was hypothesized to be higher for faculty that perceived the environment/offender to be dangerous or a threat, providing a consideration of perceived dangerousness (proximity to offender).

The study looked at both property and personal victimization that occurred among full-time faculty members at a large urban campus over a period of one year (Wooldredge et al., 1992). Demographic variables included gender, race, and age. A self-administered questionnaire was mailed with a response rate of 51%. The total sample size was 422. While support was shown for routine activities theory, there were some differences between personal and property victimization. The findings showed that for property crime, all of the guardianship variables were significant, whereas none of the guardianship variables were found to be significant for personal crime. As for the exposure variables, only one was significant for property crime (working nights and weekends), whereas three were significant for personal crime (working nights and weekends, alone on campus, and mingling with students outside of class). As for the target attractiveness variable, it was found to be insignificant for both personal and property crime. Perceived dangerousness was significant for both personal and property victimization, but was a stronger predictor for personal crimes. The demographic variables were not found to be significant for either personal or property victimization.

Overall, this study showed support for activity variables as a predictor of victimization, as opposed to demographic variables, which were not a significant predictor. In addition, domain-specific studies, such as this one, seem to better support routine activities theory and provide a better explanation of victimization.

## Property v. Personal Crime

While routine activities may aid in explaining property crime victimization, some have argued that it does not do an adequate job explaining violent crime victimization (Miethe et al., 1987). Much of the previous research testing routine activities theory has been based solely on explaining property crime (Bennett, 1991; Cohen & Cantor, 1980; Cohen et al., 1981; Massey et al., 1989; Miethe et al., 1987). However, many of these studies, while focusing on property crime, did not necessarily rule out the ability to explain violent crime.

In a 1980 study, Cohen and Cantor analyzed National Crime Survey data for 1975-76 in order to examine the characteristics of people and their lifestyles and how they may be related to the risk of larceny victimization. The variables race, age, income, major activity, and number of persons residing in the household were considered. The findings were consistent with routine activities theory. Risk of victimization was higher for those who were young, lived alone, and were either unemployed or had a higher income. Conversely, risk of victimization was lower for those who were older, earned a lower income, and whose major activity was maintaining the home.

In research conducted by Cohen et al. (1981), the findings were also consistent with routine activities theory. National Crime Survey data for 1973-74 and 1976-77 were used to determine the relationship between lifestyle and sociodemographic characteristics and the risk of being robbed. The same variables were used as in the Cohen and Cantor (1980) study. Risk of victimization was higher for those who lived in an urban area, were 29 or younger, unemployed, and unmarried. Conversely, risk of victimization was lower for those who lived in a rural area, were 30 or older, employed or retired, and married.

In a study by Massey et al. (1989), only limited support was found for a routine activities approach in the explanation of property crime. Using the 1979 Greenberg study, data from six urban neighborhoods were collected via a household survey. Three victimization measures were constructed, including a crimes against the home index (which included residential break-ins and vandalism), a theft of property index (automobile and household theft), and a total property victimization index (summation of four types of victimization) (Massey et al., 1989). Measures were also generated for the three constructs of motivated offenders, suitable targets, and guardianship. The construct of potential offenders was actually substituted for motivated offenders, as the researchers made the argument that it is a better measure—both objectively and subjectively. As such, witnessing crime, neighborhood crime, and neighborhood safety were all used as the measures for potential offenders. Target suitability was measured by housing type and security. Age and race were also included in the measure of target suitability. Guardianship was measured by whether or not someone was home during the day and weeknights. Employment, marital status, friends and relatives in the neighborhood, neighbors' help, neighbors watching home, and numbers of adults in the home were all used as measures of guardianship.

Measures of neighborhood crime, housing type, and employment status were the key determinants of risk of property crime victimization. However, none of the findings were significant, as the routine activities theory explanation of property victimization was weak at best. As for the demographic variables, some support was shown for the effects of race and age on the likelihood of property victimization. The findings indicated that being black or younger increased one's risk of victimization.

While strong support was not shown, Massey et al. (1989) suggested that future research examining individual patterns of victimization should focus on what people do to increase or decrease the chances that they will be victimized.

> Assessing the role of the victim in the explanation of crime represents an interesting and perhaps very promising line of inquiry in criminological theory construction. Yet, if victimization cannot be predicted by the steps individuals take to protect themselves and their property, the prospects for developing a sophisticated perspective on routine activities and criminal victimization will not be very promising. (Massey et al., 1989, p. 389)

In a study that examined both property and personal victimization, Miethe et al. (1987) suggested that while there is a relationship between the demographic characteristics of victims and their routine activities, it is applicable to property crime only. Using 1975 data from the National Crime Survey that was based on 107,678 residents in thirteen U.S. cities, the researchers examined rates of victimization for both property and violent crimes. Their hypothesis was that violent crime is spontaneous and therefore cannot be explained via a routine activities approach, as the rationality component is missing.

In constructing loglinear models, Miethe et al. (1987) found a relationship between certain demographic variables and risk of victimization. Specifically, single, young, poor males were at an increased risk of violent victimization. These findings were similar to those of other studies (Cohen et al., 1981; Cohen & Felson, 1979; Hindelang et al., 1978; Hindelang, 1976). When the routine activities variables were added (major activity and nighttime activity), a better fitting model was produced (Miethe et al., 1987). However, the routine activities variables did not reduce the strength of the demographic variables. While persons who participated in more nighttime activities had a greater chance of violent victimization than those who participated in fewer activities at night, there appeared to be no significant differences found between the types of major routine activities. Major routine activities referred to whether or not the activities were performed inside (homemaker, retired, unemployed, unable to work) or outside the home (work, school). Miethe et al. (1987) argued that there should be a difference depending on the type of activities in which one is engaged, whether they be at work, school, or at home. This rationale is based on the fact that suitable targets and guardianship will vary according to the activity, which seems consistent with domain-specific analyses (Lynch, 1987).

When property crime was examined, the results were different. Demographic influences suggested that property victimization was higher among households headed by young, black, single males with a higher income. When the routine activities variables were added, a better fitting model was again produced as the variables were found to be significant. Furthermore, when the routine activities variables were added, the effects of many of the demographic variables were decreased in significance and magnitude. This was consistent with previous research that explained property crime using routine activities theory (Cohen et al., 1981; Cohen & Cantor, 1980; Hindelang, 1976).

The findings of this study (Miethe et al., 1987) are contradictory to those of the Massey et al. (1989) study discussed previously. Differences in the findings may be the result of the samples used. Miethe et al. (1987) used a representative national survey, whereas Massey et al. (1989) used a neighborhood sample. In addition, the demographics of the two samples were inherently different. For example, race was used in both studies as a demographic variable; however, Miethe et al.'s sample was 70% white, in contrast to Massey et al.'s sample, which was 70% black. This may have had a bearing on the dissimilar findings.

Other studies, too, have produced contradictory findings to the Miethe et al. (1987) study. For example, some research suggests that particular lifestyles result in exposure, which creates opportunity for personal crime to occur (Kennedy & Forde, 1990). It also appears that some demographic groups are more at risk of personal victimization than others. In a study conducted by Kennedy and Forde (1990), the 1984 Canadian Urban Victimization Study was utilized. The sample of 74,463 was obtained via telephone surveys conducted among households located in seven major urban centers in Canada. Using the data, Kennedy and Forde (1990) explained personal victimization by including the amount of exposure that people experienced due to living a particular lifestyle. Furthermore, such lifestyle routines seemed to cultivate the use of certain conflict styles. Thus, the situation and the person or persons who interface with the victim appeared to unite to produce criminal opportunities. In this manner, routine activities theory may explain victimization not limited to property crime.

Messner and Tardiff (1985) also generated support for explaining personal victimization using routine activities theory. They found that age, sex, race, employment, and marital status were important indicators. In addition, temporal factors (time of day, season, and day of week) were also significant, as they reflected the geographical proximity to the victim's household and to the social proximity of participants. The sample for this study consisted of 578 homicide victims located in an urban area. The location of the homicide was found to be significantly associated with the sex, age, and employment status of the victim. The likely relationship between the offender and the victim was associated with race and sex. All of the significant associations were consistent with routine activities theory. The temporal factors were less significant, but in line with the theory. Their suggestions for future research were that categories should be less broad and more refined. For example, rather than using the broad categories of unemployed versus employed, the lifestyle activities of individuals may be better specified, such as the daily routines of the employed person versus the unemployed person.

In a study conducted by Ehrhardt-Mustaine (1999), support was found for routine activities theory as an explanation for stalking victimization among women. Surveys were given to 861 women in nine universities, comprised of both large and small institutions. While the role of demographics and statuses are often used as predictors, this study also utilized substance use variables, residence (on or off campus), and activities in public settings as predictors. The findings indicated that the risk of victimization increased for those women who used drugs and/or alcohol, lived off campus, and conducted many activities in a public setting. When these variables were introduced, the strength of the demographic and status variables was reduced.

Also, Rodgers and Roberts (1995) found limited support for using routine activities in explaining women's non-spousal multiple victimization. The findings showed little support for utilizing proximity, exposure, and guardianship variables, and found that demographic variables as predictors were not decreased when routine activities variables were added. However, the data utilized in this research were different from the Ehrhardt-Mustaine (1999) study. Rodger and Roberts (1995) used data from Canada, the Violence Against Women Survey, as opposed to the smaller, nine-institution sample used in Ehrhardt-Mustaine's (1999) study.

In research conducted by Kennedy and Silverman (1990), elderly victims of homicide were examined and routine activities theory was employed to explain this violent victimization. Using Canadian homicide statistics compiled between 1961 and 1983, the authors studied 9,642 homicide incidents involving 10,627 victims. Specifically, they considered the routine activities of the elderly and the incidences of theft-based versus non-theft based homicide. The elderly comprised approximately 8% of the total number of homicides.

The initial findings were not consistent with routine activities theory. Based on the data, it was found that the elderly were disproportionately victims of theft-based homicide. This runs contrary to routine activities theory, which would purport that because the elderly are more apt to stay at home, there would be increased guardianship. According to the propositions of routine activities theory, Kennedy and Silverman (1990) purport that "self-isolation decreases victimization, particularly theft...further, greater association with family members versus others decreases theft victimization...thus, the elderly, alone in their homes, should be relatively safe from crimes of theft and of violence (unless family members are the perpetrators)" (p. 308).

However, once the concepts were reformulated to take into account the activities of the elderly, support for the theory was found. "Interpretations of routine activities have emphasized the activities of both offender and victim that generate the crime situation...for the elderly, the routine activity is to stay at home...in other words, the activity is inactivity—a state not generally considered by the routine activity theorists" (Kennedy & Silverman, 1990, p. 308). In other words, isolation is a liability in this case, and does not necessarily decrease one's risk of victimization. The vulnerability of the elderly in their home appears to create a more attractive target.

> From this altered perspective, routine activities theory might now consider that the elderly person is not the target of the crime, but the dwelling and its contents...routine activities theory could predict that the elderly person, living quietly alone in an area with low daytime occupancy, is not detected by the burglar, or if so, is not a threat because of perceived vulnerability...in a confrontation, the elderly individual, is alone, may resist or not but is beaten...while a younger person might recover, the elderly victim dies...thus for the elderly, the safety of the home is offset by the vulnerability to attack during a crime and the difficulty in recovery from beating. (Kennedy & Silverman, 1990, p. 308)

Thus, considering the specific activities of the elderly population, including their inactivity, may increase the explanatory power of routine activities theory. This reformulation aids in the explanation of the previous inconsistent findings concerning the elderly and theft-based homicides.

Another study examined the victimization patterns of injection drug users (McElrath & Chitwood, 1997). The researchers used routine activities theory to explain both property and violent crimes among these individuals. Utilizing a sample of 308 injection drug users, the findings were consistent with routine activities theory, in that the drug user's lifestyle activity resulted in an increased risk of both property and violent victimization. Similar to other research findings (Miethe & Meier, 1990), age and gender were also found to be significant predictors of victimization.

Using data from two National Crime Survey projects—a survey of eight cities and a survey of the five largest U.S. cities—Miethe, Stafford, and Sloane (1990) extended previous routine activities research by looking at whether lifestyle changes are related to changes in a person's risk of victimization (both property and personal). The demographic variables of age, gender, and race were also included. In general, the findings were mixed. However, people taking the most precautions were not found to have the lowest risk of victimization.

When questions focus on the dynamics of change over time, routine activity/lifestyle theories may be appropriate only at the aggregate level of analysis. Changes in lifestyle that decrease guardianship and enhance exposure to crime do not necessarily lead to increased risks of victimization for individuals. The importance of these findings should not be underestimated because they are clearly contrary to routine activity/lifestyle theories as currently stated. At the very least, these theories seem to need some modification when applied to changes in individuals' risks of victimization over time. Nonetheless, the association between change and stability in lifestyles and criminal victimization suggests that much may be learned about the social ecology of crime from a more systematic investigation of changes in the routine activities and opportunity structure of everyday life. (Miethe et al., 1990, p. 374)

However, it should be noted that because of the data utilized, measures of neighborhood characteristics were not available, which may have had a bearing on the findings. The data collected from the two National Crime Surveys was also limited in that information could only be provided from the questions that were asked. Specifically, the surveys asked about routine activities in terms of major daytime and nighttime activity patterns, household composition, as well as the number of places avoided or activities limited due to fear of crime. In addition, determining passive and active lifestyle changes were also subject to the types of questions asked in the original surveys. For example, there was difficulty in determining whether or not precautionary measures were taken before or after the victimization, due to the way the questions were worded on the survey. "The distinction between passive and active lifestyle changes is important because victimization risks may be as strongly influenced by changes in routine activities that are not undertaken explicitly to reduce victimization risks as by conscious efforts to minimize them" (Miethe et al., 1990, p. 373).

The findings indicated that passive lifestyle changes were more important than active lifestyle changes. However, the impact of those passive changes was not the same across the board for both personal and property victimization. "For example, the impact of changes in activity outside the household varied somewhat by type of crime and whether it was a daytime or nighttime activity, whereas the effects of guardianship were fairly similar across crime categories and equally predictive of different types of transitions in victimization status" (Miethe et al., 1990, p. 374). A question for future research would be whether or not the impact of passive lifestyle changes on risk of victimization would be the same in different environments, considering both high and low crime neighborhoods, or would active lifestyle changes prove to be more significant to victimization risk. Since the data were not available on the characteristics of the neighborhoods in which the surveys were conducted, this could not be determined from the study.

In sum, while some research discussed above indicates that routine activities best explains property crime as opposed to personal crime, such findings may have much to do with the data employed. In addition, how one measures the routine activities variables also has a strong bearing on the findings. For example, Kennedy and Forde (1990) found support for routine activities theory in explaining violent victimization as well as property victimization. While the findings for property victimization were similar to those found in the Miethe et al. (1987) study, the findings for personal victimization were quite different. Kennedy and Forde (1990) used data from a survey that contained detailed measures of routine activities, which was not available in the study conducted by Miethe et al. (1987). Kennedy and Forde's (1990) research considered more details about individuals' different activities, while Miethe et al. (1987) used composite measures of routine activities. Also, the data used in the Kennedy and Forde (1990) study provided additional detail about criminal victimization, which the Miethe et al. (1987) data set did not contain.

## Integrating Other Theories

Other studies have attempted to increase the explanatory power of routine activities theory in explaining violent crime by integrating or adding other theoretical components. For example, Kennedy and Baron (1993) conducted a qualitative study utilizing both the routine activities and subcultural approaches. While previous research utilizing routine activities theory typically suggested a correlation between personal and property victimization and lifestyle patterns/degree of exposure, Kennedy and Baron (1993) proposed that integrating routine activities theory with a subcultural approach and incorporating a choice component would strengthen the explanatory power. They argued that routine activities theory, by itself, does not sufficiently explain how interactions give rise to violence. Rather, "subcultural norms influence actors' routine activities that, in turn, influence exposure to victimization and shape the behavioral choices available to members in response to victimization" (Kennedy & Baron, 1993, p. 88).

Based on the interviews, the authors found an emerging theme. The study examined a delinquent street gang and the subcultural norms that guided their behavior. In this case, the value of violence among gang members was examined. While it appeared that violence was valued among gang members, the authors found that some had never been involved in violence. The authors derived three primary explanations from their research: opportunity, status, and fear. First, some of the situations that may have resulted in a violent incident occurred on busy streets, which in turn limited the opportunity to react violently. Second, some of the situations occurred at times and places where other gang members were not present, thereby eliminating the possibility for that member to receive sanctions or status from the rest of the group. Last, members who feared being victimized would change their behavior accordingly. For example, gang members who feared victimization rarely would go out without being accompanied by other gang members.

Based on the authors' research, it appeared that subcultural norms do influence routine activities, which subsequently influenced the situations and conditions in which violence may occur. Thus, the authors concluded that a choice component should be added, as the likelihood of violence occurring is dependent on the rational choices that the gang members make in those situations. Furthermore, the authors conclude that the subcultural literature should be consulted in order to determine "how conflict styles mediate the impact of exposure to high-risk situations" (Kennedy & Baron, 1993, p. 112).

Other studies have also shown support for a subcultural element or demographic variations (Jensen & Brownfield, 1986; Kennedy & Forde, 1990; Sampson & Wooldredge, 1987). For example, there has been a correlation established between frequenting bars or drinking establishments and victimization (Kennedy & Forde, 1990; Lasley, 1989). According to Jensen and Brownfield (1986), certain routines may be of a criminogenic nature, thus increasing the likelihood for victimization. Furthermore, individual lifestyle patterns may not increase the likelihood of more contact with potential offenders, but rather certain activities may have a relationship with deviant behavior itself. Thus, the likelihood of personal victimization increases among those who engage in deviant or criminal activities themselves. Moreover, offender and victim characteristics may reflect this commonality. "The lifestyles that lead one to bar behavior and to being on the street lead to situations in which these factors coincide to present offenders with opportunities to commit crime" (Kennedy & Baron, 1993, p. 91).

On the other hand, some routine activities research suggests that an increase in victimization may occur regardless of the cultural or structural conditions that may motivate persons to commit crime (Lauritsen et al., 1991; Sampson & Lauritsen, 1990). Sampson and Lauritsen (1990) argued that the likelihood of being victimized increases with the amount of contact a person has with groups of people who are known to commit a disproportionate amount of crime. For example, the mentally ill as a group appear to commit a disproportionate amount of crime (Monahan, 1992). Thus, one could make the argument that mental health workers would be at a greater risk because of their contact with this population, although they are not engaging in deviant behavior themselves.

Along these same lines, although support has been shown for subcultural norms having an influence on routine activities and thus the situations in which violence may occur, the populations studied were also more apt or prone to become involved in deviant behavior. For example, Kennedy and Baron's (1993) study examined victimization among delinquent street gangs, Jensen and Brownfield's (1986) research examined victimization among female students, and Finkelhor & Asdigian (1996) also looked at youth victimization, as adolescents are extremely vulnerable to victimization (Finkelhor & Ormrod, 1999). From such studies it is often difficult to determine which came first, the engagement in delinquent behavior or the victimization.

## Micro v. Macro-Level Explanations

"Recent research has emphasized the complementary nature of macro-social (group, contextual, or aggregate) and micro (individual-level) factors in the explanation of variation in crime and delinquency" (Rountree et al., 1994, p. 387). Typically, routine activities theory has been presented as a macro-level perspective examining the effects of urban structure on crime rates (Cao & Maume, 1993; Chamlin & Cochran, 1994; Cohen & Felson, 1979; Felson & Cohen, 1980; Parker & Toth, 1990). Routine activities theory has been able to explain patterns of urban victimization, with fairly strong predictive capabilities (Kennedy & Forde, 1990). Such macro-level studies have generally relied upon large-scale victimization surveys or police statistics (Schwartz & Pitts, 1995).

Other studies have tested routine activities theory from a micro-level perspective. Micro-level predictions, however, have not been as strong or robust (Miethe et al., 1987; Sampson & Wooldredge, 1987). For example, in one study, routine activities adequately explained property crime, but not personal crime (Miethe et al., 1987). In another study, demographics and structural characteristics were found to be more significant in explaining crime than were particular lifestyle activities (Sampson & Wooldredge, 1987). In yet another piece of research, both individual and group-level variables were found to be important indicators of property crime (Kennedy & Forde, 1990). Furthermore, while urban structure had an impact on personal crimes, it was best explained using individual-level variables.

However, micro-level analyses utilizing routine activities variables have revealed predictability in some research (Schwartz & Pitts, 1995; Wooldredge et al., 1992). This may be due, in part, to the type of methods used. For example, Schwartz and Pitts (1995) conducted a victimization study examining the relationship between drinking and sexual assault. In looking at sexual assaults on college campuses, they distributed questionnaires to a sample of 288 undergraduate females from an urban campus. Support was found for using routine activities variables and feminist theory in the explanation of campus sexual assault. On the other hand, had a large-scale victimization survey been conducted, support may not have been found due to reporting differences. Women's reporting rates of sexual crimes are still low, and thus such a problem may be poorly measured. Thus, while there is still the chance that women may not report such victimization to researchers, smaller-scale victimization surveys may yield better results.

## Summary

In reviewing the literature, there has been substantial empirical research on routine activities theory (Cohen & Felson, 1979). Routine activities theory has been used in domain-specific research, utilized in the explanation of both property and violent victimization, integrated with other theories, and used on both a micro and macro level. While some of the research has provided further empirical support for the theory and has examined a wide range of phenomena, there does appear to be some limitations and areas that merit more research.

Limitations of prior research pertain to the types of data used, the measurement of routine activities concepts, and the use of generalized models. For example, much of the past research has relied on household victimization surveys and official crime statistics (Kennedy & Baron, 1993; Sherman et al., 1989). Furthermore, over-reliance on demographic variables as measures of key concepts has also been criticized (Miethe et al., 1987). Relying on demographic variables to infer routine activities patterns raises questions with regard to construct validity. It has been suggested that the measurement of the three key concepts—motivated offenders, suitable targets, and guardianship—should be more narrowly defined, thus providing more accurate measures (Lynch, 1987). In doing so, the use of domain-specific models should be utilized in favor of generalized models. In addition, all three concepts should be included in empirical tests, including the concept of motivated offenders. Previous research has virtually ignored the concept of motivated offenders by making the assumption that it is a constant motivation for all persons (Bryant & Miller, 1997; Massey et al., 1989; Miethe et al., 1987; Osgood et al., 1996; Schwartz & Pitts, 1995; Sutton, 1995).

While routine activities theory has been substantively tested since its conception, there are still areas in which additional research is needed. While there has been some testing of routine activities theory using domain-specific victimization models, there has been less research attention given to the specific domain of the workplace and certain high-risk workplaces. While the purpose of the present study was to provide a test of routine activities theory using a domain-specific victimization model, the study also provided descriptive data regarding violence that occurs in the mental health workplace. The next chapter examines what we do know about violence in the workplace, as well as current ideas on the connection between mental illness and violence.

# CHAPTER II

# Violence in the Workplace

Block, Felson, and Block (1984) are credited for their early work that examined victimization in the workplace. The data were collected from nine National Crime Surveys, which included over two million respondents during the years of 1973 through 1981. The authors concluded, "occupations may be seen as routine activities which structure daily life, hence exposing people and property to risk of attack by offenders" (Block et al., 1984, p. 442). The findings were based on 1,330 occupation-specific rates of victimization and were obtained through a two-equation model focusing on income and urbanization. Specifically, urbanization was positively correlated with risk of victimization, while higher income positions reduced the risk of victimization. The results were consistent for five crimes: robbery, assault, burglary, larceny, and auto theft. Other subsequent studies examined the relationship between victimization and particular occupations (NIOSH, 1993a; NIOSH 1993b; Warchol, 1998). Southerland et al. (1997) credited a 1993 study conducted by the National Institute for Occupational Safety and Health (NIOSH) and data collected by the United States Bureau of Labor Statistics as the primary sources of information about this problem.

More recently, the National Crime Victimization Survey found that between 1992 and 1996, over two million violent victimizations occurred each year in the United States to persons while they were at work (Warchol, 1998). On average, 14.8 victimizations were experienced per 1000 workers. Simple assaults comprised a majority of the victimizations. Other studies conducted have focused primarily on the setting in which the violence occurs, various environmental and situational factors, and the individual traits of the victims, offenders, or both.

## Setting

Four main types of violence have been identified, based on research that focuses on the work setting in which violent acts are carried out and the actors involved (Capozzoli and McVey, 1996; Lester & Maccone, 2001; Peek-Asa et al., 1998). The first type involves violence that begins and occurs in the workplace (Capozzoli & McVey, 1996). Typically, this involves employee-on-employee violence and may include both former and current employees (Peek-Asa et al., 1998). However, this may also include current or past customers, clients or patients as well. For example, a hospitalized patient in a treatment setting may assault a nurse, or a client residing in a group home may assault a counselor. Studies have shown that certain workplace environments have become increasingly dangerous (Anderson & Stamper, 2001; Carroll, 1996; Hoag-Apel, 1998; Racette, 2001; Sullivan & Yuan, 1995; Warshaw & Messite, 1996). For instance, hospital emergency rooms and health care facilities have been witnessing violence by former clients and patients. A study conducted in Los Angeles County found that health care workers (general and mental health) had higher victimization rates in the workplace compared to other county employees (Sullivan & Yuan, 1995).

The second type involves violence that starts in the workplace, but then occurs outside of the workplace (Capozzoli & McVey, 1996). For example, a disgruntled employee may take action against another employee or supervisor outside of work. This type of violence is not limited to employees or former employees, as it may also include assaults by customers, patients, or clients as well (Lester & Maccone, 2001; Peek-Asa et al., 1998). For instance, a disappointed or unhappy client might take action in retaliation against an employee outside of the workplace.

The third type involves violence that begins outside of the workplace but is eventually brought into the workplace (Capozzoli & McVey, 1996). The disturbing events that took place on September 11, 2001 are examples of how violence may be brought into the workplace

(Lester & Maccone, 2001). The 1995 bombing of the federal building in Oklahoma City would also be a case of violence brought into the workplace in the course of criminal activity (Nigro & Waugh, 1996). Less high-profile cases would include robberies committed by nonemployees or strangers (Lester & Maccone, 2001; Peek-Asa et al., 1998). Convenience stores and service stations may provide an environment that is conducive to violence, especially by strangers (Capozzoli & McVey, 1996). In fact, National Crime Victimization Survey data from 1992 to 1996 showed that robbery was the cause of most workplace homicides (Warchol, 1998).

The last type includes violence by an intimate partner or precipitated by a love interest (Lester & Maccone, 2001; Peek-Asa et al., 1998). For example, domestic violence may spill over into the workplace (Capozzoli & McVey, 1996; Carroll, 2000; Labig, 1995; Lester & Maccone, 2001; Moffatt, 1998; NIOSH, 1993a; NIOSH, 1993b). One study found that violence by an intimate partner constituted 5% of the total workplace victimizations (NIOSH, 1996). According to Capozzoli and McVey (1996), statistics show that family violence is increasing in the United States and may also be contributing to more incidences of workplace violence. In addition to domestic violence spillovers, acts of stalking and sexual harassment also add to the problem of violence in the workplace (Moffatt, 1998).

When defining what acts constitute workplace violence, they should not be limited to the confines of the workplace, as they may not necessarily occur in the workplace environment itself. Rather, acts of violence may originate in the workplace but subsequently be carried out elsewhere. Conversely, violence may also be brought into the workplace. Upon examination of specific types of workplace settings, violence is not equally or randomly distributed. According to NIOSH (1996), violence in the workplace is found in clusters in particular settings. In general, workplace violence incidences are more likely to occur in private companies as opposed to the public sector (NIOSH, 1996). It is estimated that only 30% of victimizations in the workplace occur in the public sector (Nigro & Waugh, 1996). The highest rates of violence have been found in retail trade and service industries (i.e. grocery stores, restaurants/bars, taxi services) and public order/justice establishments (LaMar, Gerberich, Lohman, & Zaidman, 1998; Nigro & Waugh, 1996; NIOSH, 1993a; NIOSH, 1993b; NIOSH, 1996).

## Environmental & Situational Factors

Specific situational and environmental factors have been cited frequently in the literature as having a positive correlation with risk of victimization in the workplace (LaMar et al., 1998; Nigro & Waugh, 1996; NIOSH, 1993a; NIOSH, 1993b; NIOSH, 1996; Warshaw & Messite, 1996). They include the following: working and exchanging money with the public; delivering passengers, services, or goods; guarding possessions or property of great value; carrying drugs or having access to drugs; conducting work in a mobile place (i.e., taxi or patrol car); working solely or in small groups; working particular hours or shifts (i.e., late at night or during early morning); working with capricious individuals (i.e., those in health care, social service, or criminal justice settings); carrying out inspection procedures; working in crime-prone areas; and working in community-based settings.

The environment in which one works also plays a role in the risk of victimization. For example, in looking at the field of mental health, "the risk varies with the environment: hospitalized patients, even though they tend to be more severely ill, are perhaps less likely to be violent because of the supervision, care, medication, and support they receive, as compared with those who have been deinstitutionalized and must cope with the stresses of living at home and in the community" (Warshaw & Messite, 1996, p. 996). Thus, mentally ill clients or patients may pose more of a risk when visiting an outpatient clinic or emergency room, or receiving at-home visits, as compared to being confined at a hospital. Therefore, depending on the workplace setting, employees may also be more at risk.

## Individual Traits

On an individual level, factors or causes have been identified that play a role in the likelihood of a violent episode occurring in the workplace (Baron & Neuman, 1996; Calabrese, 2000; Capozzoli & McVey, 1996; Hlebovy, 2000; Jockin, Arvey, & McGue, 2001; Kline & Sussman, 2000; Labig, 1995; Laschinger, Finegan, & Shamian, 2001; Nigro & Waugh, 1996; Warshaw & Messite, 1996). The threat of losing one's job or a threat to one's person is a factor and may include: a poor working environment, possible downsizing, lack of support and participation in the decision-making process, role ambiguity or role conflict. Other factors such as mental illness, substance abuse, family and marital problems, and nonspecific stress have also been cited as contributing to violence in the workplace. Because the current study focuses on the risk of victimization among mental health workers, the role of mental illness will be discussed further. For general reviews of the literature regarding the other factors, consult Capozzoli & McVey (1996) and Labig (1995).

## Role of Mental Illness

Since this study examined victimization that occurs in the workplace among mental health workers, a review of the literature surrounding the relationship between mental illness and violence is warranted. Upon examination of the literature, there appears to be some controversy as to the risk that the mentally ill pose to others (Appelbaum et al., 2000; Baron & Neuman, 1996; Capozzoli & McVey, 1996; Labig, 1995; Laden & Schwartz, 2000; Monahan & Arnold, 1996; Nigro & Waugh, 1996; Steinert, 2001; Warshaw & Messite, 1996). However, the weight of the literature suggests that there is a connection between mental illness and violence (Arango, Barba, Gonzalez-Salvador, & Ordonez, 1999; Arseneault et al., 2000; Bartels, Drake, Wallach, & Freeman, 1991; Eronen et al., 1996; Hodgins, 1992; Hodgins et al., 1996; Kasper, Hoge, Feucht-Haviar, Cortina, & Cohen, 1997; Lindqvist & Allebeck, 1990; Link et al., 1992; Link et al., 1999; Martell & Dietz, 1992; Marzuk, 1996; Modestin & Ammann, 1996; Monahan, 1992; Rabkin, 1979; Rasanen, Tiihonen, Isohanni, Rantakallio, Lehtonen, & Moring, 1998; Shore et al., 1990; Smith, 1989; Sosowsky, 1980; Swanson et al., 1997; Swanson et al., 1990; Swartz et al., 1998; Taylor, 1985; Taylor, Leese, Williams, Butwell, Daly, & Larkin, 1998; Wessely, Castle, Douglas, & Taylor, 1994). This correlation has been shown using different types of samples and research methodologies.

For example, longitudinal studies that examine patients' behaviors after treatment have shown a significant level of violence on the part of the mentally ill (Eronen et al., 1996; Hodgins, 1992; Hodgins et al., 1996; Lindqvist & Allebeck, 1990; Link et al., 1992; Monahan, 1992; Rabkin, 1979; Shore et al., 1990; Sosowsky, 1980; Swanson et al., 1990; Swanson et al., 1997; Swartz et al., 1998). Furthermore, the research suggests that there are much higher rates of violence among the mentally ill, as compared to the general population. To illustrate, between the years 1972 and 1978, arrest rates for 301 patients discharged from a California state hospital were compared to the arrest rates for those in the local county (Sosowsky, 1980). The researcher examined both the arrest rates of patients before hospitalization and after their release. The follow-up period varied in time for patients depending on their release date. The arrest rate for the comparison group was taken for the last year of the follow-up period (1978). The findings showed that the violent crime arrest rate of discharged patients was five times greater than that of the general population. Ex-patients with no previous arrests prior to hospitalization were found to have an arrest rate three times greater than the general population. While the findings clearly indicated that violent crime arrest rates were higher for ex-patients than the general population, it is not known if the comparison group's arrest rate was higher or lower than the average arrest rate for the six-year period, as the arrest rate for the comparison group was only taken for 1978. Overall, the comparability of the two groups is in question.

Swanson et al. (1990) reported that Epidemiological Catchment Area (ECA) surveys conducted in the early 1980s also indicated that persons with severe mental illness exhibited higher rates of violence as compared to other community members. Based on self-reports, the researchers surveyed approximately 10,000 respondents in three metropolitan areas. The Diagnostic Interview Schedule (DIS) was utilized in order to generate DSM-III diagnoses. The DIS is a structured interview schedule and was administered by trained lay persons. The diagnoses included in this study were major depression, mania, panic, obsessive-compulsive and bipolar disorder, schizophrenia, alcohol and drug abuse or dependence, and phobia. In order to qualify under DSM-III, respondents had to have met the criteria for a disorder within the preceding twelve months of the interview. The DIS also included five items relating to violent behavior. To qualify as having committed a violent act, the act must have been committed during the twelve months preceding the interview. A one-year time period was chosen because both lesser or greater time periods may have resulted in an underestimation of the problem. For example, violence may not have manifested itself during a six-month period, or violence may not have been adequately recalled during a three-year period. In both cases, an inadequate picture of violence may be presented. Of course, underreporting is always an issue with self-reports as they may underestimate the problem as well.

Analysis of the ECA surveys found that persons with psychiatric disorders were more likely to commit violence than those who did not have a mental disorder and were not afflicted with drug and alcohol abuse. Additionally, having both a mental illness and a substance abuse problem resulted in a greater propensity towards violence. "One could say that the combination of substance abuse with other major psychopathology is more volatile than either alone" (Swanson et al., 1990, p. 768). The researchers also found that the likelihood of violence increased with the number of psychiatric diagnoses a person had received.

Other research has shown that a failure to treat mental illness results in high rates of violence (Bartels et al., 1991; Kasper et al., 1997; Martell & Dietz, 1992; Smith, 1989; Swartz et al., 1998; Taylor, 1985). For example, Kasper et al. (1997) studied 348 patients at a state psychiatric hospital over a six-month period and found that those who failed to take prescribed medications were more likely to be violent. Using the Brief Psychiatric Rating Scale (BPRS), surveys were given to newly admitted patients about their attitudes toward admission. The BPRS contained nineteen questions and was administered by psychiatrists. The interviews were carried out within the first day of admission. Patients who refused medication at the time of admittance were compared to a group of patients who were compliant. The findings suggested that those who were noncompliant were negative, more likely to be assaultive, and required lengthier hospitalization stays as compared to compliant patients.

In another study, Bartels et al. (1991) examined a sample of 133 outpatients followed over a six-month period and found that 13% were characterized as violent, 18% as threatening, and 21% as argumentative and irritable. Forty-eight percent were classified as having no hostility. Follow-ups over a one-year period revealed that hostility was predictive of subsequent hospitalization. All of the subjects for this study were involved with the Ambulatory Community Service (i.e., or assertive case management), which is a mobile, multidisciplinary unit of community-based therapists who provide outpatient services to patients discharged from the state hospital. All patients in the sample received such services because they were identified as having a severe illness.

While only a small proportion of the sample exhibited violent behaviors, the findings also suggested that those who were more hostile were more likely to abuse drugs and alcohol. Fifty-nine percent of the patients rated as violent also had a substance abuse problem.

Martel and Dietz (1992) also found similar results. The researchers studied twenty people who had pushed or attempted to push a person in front of a subway car. The data about the offenders were obtained from records kept by the Bureau of Forensic Services of the New York State Office of Mental Health, which included police, criminal and mental health treatment records, and court documents. Nineteen out of twenty were found to have severe mental illness. Their motives for the act were linked to their untreated mental illness, as 95% of the perpetrators were psychotic when the act occurred. It should be noted that the researchers originally identified 41 persons who were involved in pushing or attempting to push others onto subway tracks between the years 1975 and 1991. Of which, 36 acted alone, and five were in groups. The five acting in groups appeared connected to gang violence, of which one was referred to treatment. Of the 36 individuals, not all were referred to psychiatric evaluation. The researchers deliberately selected 20 of the individuals who were referred to treatment in order to examine the characteristics of the offenders.

While the authors state that violent acts such as these are uncommon and often sensationalized in the media, they do make the argument that an increase in such incidences is positively correlated with an increase in mentally ill persons living in an area and an increase in the number of homeless individuals, as 65% of the offenders were homeless at the time the incident occurred. However, the sample size was relatively small, and included only acts that were reported. The sample did not include unreported attempts. This may have resulted in findings that do not paint an accurate picture of the problem and the characteristics of the offenders.

Another group of studies have examined the mental illness-violence connection by considering varying types of mental illness (Arango et al., 1999; Link et al., 1992; Modestin & Ammann, 1996; Taylor et al., 1998; Wessely et al., 1994). For example, Wessely et al. (1994) studied 538 schizophrenics and found that these men and women posed a greater risk for committing violent acts than did those in the comparison groups (i.e., persons with other psychiatric diagnoses). The cohort study was based on schizophrenic individuals identified from a community psychiatric case register. The case register provided a comprehensive list of all individuals diagnosed with schizophrenia between the years 1965 and 1984 in that designated geographic area. Clinical case records of the 538 identified were obtained in order to provide further information. Data were collected on the subjects' medical conditions, criminal histories, and personal information. Thus, a limitation of this study is that it only includes cases of known mental illness. Overall, the findings suggested that schizophrenic patients, compared to those with other psychiatric conditions, have an increased risk of offending. These findings are consistent with other studies that have found schizophrenia to be positively correlated with violence (Arango et al., 1999; Modestin & Ammann, 1996; Taylor et al., 1998).

In response to the debate over mental illness and violent behavior, Monahan (1992) stated:

> The data that have recently become available, fairly read, suggest the one conclusion I did not want to reach: Whether the measure is the prevalence of violence among the disordered or the prevalence of disorder among the violent, whether the sample is people who are selected for treatment as inmates or patients in institutions or people randomly chosen from the open community, and no matter how many social and demographic factors are statistically taken into account, there appears to be a relationship between mental disorder and violent behavior. (p. 519)

Along similar lines, Marzuk (1996) reported, "in the last decade, the evidence showing a link between violence, crime, and mental illness has mounted. It cannot be dismissed; it should not be ignored" (p. 481). As stated before, the weight of the literature supports the connection between mental illness and violence. As such, there are relatively fewer studies that have challenged this position.

However, some researchers suggest that the mentally ill pose no more of a threat than do other members of society arguing that the relationship between mental illness and violence is weak at best (Bower, 1998; Monahan & Arnold, 1996; Steadman et al., 1998). It has been suggested by Monahan and Arnold (1996) that the controversy over the mental illness—violence connection may have to do more with how the question is posed.

> If the question is, "Is there any relationship between major mental illness and the commission of violent behavior to others?" the answer provided by current research is, "Yes." But if the question is, "Is there a strong relationship between major mental illness and the commission of violence to others?" the answer to emerge from recent studies is equally clear, "No." (Monahan & Arnold, 1996, p. 71)

Furthermore, a recent study by the MacArthur Foundation has provided evidence that the mentally ill pose no more of a threat than any other person in the general population when substance abuse is taken into account (Steadman et al., 1998). The findings suggested that both nonpatients and discharged psychiatric patients were found to have higher rates of violence when afflicted with a substance abuse problem as compared to those who do not. The sample consisted of 951 people who had been discharged from a psychiatric facility in three metropolitan areas. The comparison group consisted of 519 people (nonpatients) selected at random from one of the three metropolitan areas. Interviews were conducted with patients every ten weeks for the year following their discharge. Interviews were conducted once with nonpatients, inquiring about their violent behavior in the past ten weeks. Additional information about both groups was obtained from friends and family of the participants as well as police and hospital records.

The proportion of patients who committed a violent act during the study year was 18% for those with a major mental disorder (such as schizophrenia or manic depression) who also showed no signs of substance abuse, 31% for patients with both a major mental disorder and substance abuse, and 43% for patients with another mental condition (such as a personality disorder) and substance abuse (Steadman et al., 1998). Nonpatients and patients not suffering from a substance abuse problem were found to have similar violence rates. In addition, the study found that the rates of violence were higher preceding hospitalization than after discharge. Furthermore, a comparison of violence rates showed an additional decrease approximately one year after discharge. However, it should be noted that this decrease may be due, in part, to the following: higher attrition rates by patients who were more violent, less time spent in the community during the follow up period (i.e., incarcerated or hospitalized), or some patients may not have disclosed violent acts actually committed.

While these results indicate that the mentally ill may be no more violent than anyone else, there appear to be some limitations to the study. First, the sample was limited to those who were discharged from acute-care hospitals. Only one in ten patients was hospitalized more than thirty days. Therefore, anyone who had been confined to a long-term psychiatric or forensic hospital, prison, or jail would not be included in the sample (Satel & Jaffe, 1998). Hence, those persons who may be the most violent were not included, resulting in a lower risk sample. Second, acts considered to be violent were limited to those that resulted in bodily harm only. By limiting the definition in this way, other acts, such as an attempt to punch or hit another, or an act resulting in property damage, would not be considered an act of violence. Third, mental illness was broadly defined, including both nonpsychotic and psychotic individuals. Thus, those suffering from depression, which constituted 40% of the sample, would seemingly be less likely to commit violence as compared to those who are schizophrenic. Last, the comparison group was selected from only one of the three cities in the study. The participants selected generally came from areas of the city that had higher rates of crime overall and were characterized as the poorer, drug-infested areas of the city, possibly leading to a control group more prone to violence, and thus a high-risk group. Given the limitations to this study, it is unclear as to whether the mentally ill—as defined by the researchers—are in fact no more violent than anyone else.

Based on the literature, there does appear to be some controversy regarding the risk of violence that the mentally ill pose in comparison to other groups. However, the weight of the evidence seems to support a positive correlation between mental illness and violence. This specific controversy is not addressed in this study, but given the current research, mental health workers may be at a higher risk of violent victimization in the workplace.

# Evaluation of the Workplace Violence Literature

One of the criticisms of the current research on workplace violence pertains to the lack of available data. The literature indicates that some aspects of workplace violence receive more attention than others. For example, while homicide represents the smallest percentage of workplace violence occurrences, it is generally the most often researched (Anderson & Stamper, 2001; Hashemi & Webster, 1998; LaMar et al., 1998). This may be attributed to another problem—reporting practices. Generally speaking, homicide is much more likely to be reported to the police than other types of crimes. Differences in reporting practices, as well as how acts of workplace violence are defined, may paint a picture that underestimates victimization in particular industries. Furthermore, the environmental and situational factors, as well as other individual traits, that have been identified were based on employees' reports of experiencing violence within the workplace. Thus, without accurate, available data, the impact of such factors and traits may not be fully understood.

Overall, there appear to be differences in reporting practices for certain industries (Peek-Asa et al., 1998). This refers to differences as to whether or not the act of violence is reported to the police or just the employer. For example, Peek-Asa et al. (1998) examined non-fatal workplace assaults and found that hospitals, police/security, and schools had higher rates of victimization than were shown by police reports. This was attributed to reporting practices among these three industries whereby employees would report the violent act directly to their employer, as opposed to reporting it to the police. In another study, Warchol (1998) found, from victimization surveys, that less than half of all nonfatal violent incidences occurring at work among health professionals were reported to the police. "When questioned about why they did not report the offense, workplace violence victims gave as their most common reason that they reported to another official" (Warchol, 1998, p. 5).

Conversely, industries such as retail stores and certain service industries are more likely to report workplace violence incidences to the police, and thus tend to have higher official rates of workplace violence (Peek-Asa et al., 1998). Such reporting discrepancies create misleading data. According to Peek-Asa et al. (1998), "surveillance of non-fatal workplace assault injuries using only one reporting source could severely underestimate incidences and fail to identify important epidemiological characteristics of these events" (p. 712). While police reports have been a valuable source of information, they appear to offer a different profile as compared to the one revealed through reports to employers. Thus, it seems necessary to include other sources of information in addition to police reports, in order to obtain a complete picture of violence in the workplace. For example, in a study conducted by Sullivan and Yuan (1995), the Los Angeles County workers compensation database was used to research nonfatal workplace assaults. In general, workers compensation reports were regarded as complete for supplying information on acute injuries that result in lost time at work or medical treatment, as the source of injury was documented.

How workplace violence is defined and measured and what receives research attention may also contribute to why certain industries appear to have higher rates of victimization than others. Current research has shown that actual rates of workplace violence may be higher than initially reported due to the way information is maintained (Nigro & Waugh, 1996; Warshaw & Messite, 1996). For example, Capozzoli and McVey (1996) state that "in the absence of a formal reporting system, complete and accurate statistics upon which to estimate total primary and secondary costs to employers and victims in an average year are nonexistent" (p. 28). Also, victimization studies have indicated that many acts of workplace violence go unreported even to the employer (Anderson & Stamper, 2001; McKoy & Smith, 2001; NIOSH, 1996; Warshaw & Messite, 1996). This may be attributed to a variety of reasons including fear, an attitude that "nothing can be done about it," a lack of a reporting system within the workplace, or the act itself not being recognized as workplace violence.

## Summary

Violence in the workplace has emerged over the last decade as a problem of significant proportion (Laden & Schwartz, 2000; NIOSH 1993a; NIOSH 1993b; Southerland et al., 1997; Warchol, 1998). With over two million violent victimizations occurring each year in the workplace (Warchol, 1998), it is a problem that warrants further research attention. A review of the literature revealed that violence may occur in a variety of settings, and the actors involved include both current and former employees, customers, patients, clients, as well as strangers and intimate partners (Capozzoli & McVey, 1996; Lester & Maccone, 2001; Peek-Asa et al., 1998). In addition, environmental and situational factors, as well as individual traits, have been identified as having a significant correlation with risk of victimization in the workplace. Since the present study examined the risk of victimization among mental health workers, the focus was on the role of mental illness. While it has been established that workplace violence is a problem, there appears to be controversy as to the role that the mentally ill play and their subsequent impact on victimization rates (Appelbaum et al., 2000; Baron & Neuman, 1996; Capozzoli & McVey, 1996; Labig, 1995; Laden & Schwartz, 2000; Monahan & Arnold, 1996; Nigro & Waugh, 1996; Steinert, 2001; Warshaw & Messite, 1996). This study did not provide information that settles this controversy, but rather provided information regarding violence and the mentally ill by probing into the perceptions of mental health workers.

In addition, this study also addressed one of the criticisms of the current research, that is, the lack of data available on workplace violence. The lack of data is attributed, in part, to how the violent incident is reported (whether it is reported to the police, employer, or another third party). It appears that there are differences in reporting practices for certain industries (Peek-Asa et al., 1998). Differences in reporting practices (i.e., whether or not an act is reported to the police) may paint a picture that underestimates victimization in particular industries. Furthermore, how an act of workplace violence is defined may also play a role in whether or not it is reported. For example, if it is not recognized as violence, it will not be reported as such. The current study addressed these issues by surveying mental health workers directly regarding their perceptions and experiences with violence in the workplace.

## The Present Study

Upon examination of the literature, few studies adequately examine the risk of victimization among mental health workers, specifically client-on-employee violence. While studies have included mental health employees among categories of various occupations and in examining the subsequent risk of victimization in a particular field, there is an absence of empirical studies that specifically and solely examine the mental health field. In addition, there is also a lack of research that utilizes routine activities theory and domain-specific victimization models to explain violence in the workplace, especially the field of mental health. By studying mental health workers only, it is possible to discover attributes of the job that play a role in victimization.

As suggested by Lynch (1987), the use of domain-specific victimization models, as opposed to generalized models, should increase explanatory power while maintaining generalizability. Wooldredge et al. (1992) concluded that "research on single occupational domains...is likely to be more rigorous than general work studies because such research makes it possible to develop very specific measures of work-related activities...[which is] useful for advancing [routine activities] theory" (p. 327). Thus, looking at a single occupation allows for the further refining of routine activities' key concepts (motivated offenders, suitable targets, and guardianship). This is important, as some routine activities research has been criticized for its poor measurement of the key concepts, especially the concept of motivated offenders (Bryant & Miller, 1997; Massey et al., 1989; Miethe et al., 1987; Osgood et al., 1996; Schwartz & Pitts, 1995; Sutton, 1995).

In this study, the concept of motivated offenders was examined critically. Sampson and Lauritsen (1990) argued that the likelihood of being victimized increases with the amount of contact a person has with groups of people who are known to commit a disproportionate amount of crime. While the mental illness – violence connection has been debated, the weight of the literature suggests that there is a positive correlation between mental illness and violence. Thus, one could make the argument that mental health workers would be at a greater risk because of their contact with this population. By surveying mental health workers directly, it may be possible to better determine the level of violence that occurs, as well as to examine perceptions about this victimization.

This study did not utilize existing data from household victimization surveys, but rather, data were obtained via individual surveys distributed to employees working in the field of mental health. In addition, preliminary interviews were conducted in order to create an improved survey instrument and to provide supplementary qualitative data. Finally, it is anticipated that the findings from this study can be utilized to improve and expand upon current prevention methods and strategies.

# CHAPTER III

# Research Methodology

The purpose of this study was to examine the relationship between the routine activities of mental health workers and their risk of violent victimization. In order to accomplish this task, a dual methodological approach was carried out. Using routine activities theory (Cohen & Felson, 1979) as a theoretical framework, the present study examined the activity patterns of mental health employees and considered how their activities may play a role in increasing or decreasing their risk of victimization. The variables employed measured the target suitability of the worker and the presence or lack of guardianship, and were used to investigate how these factors affect the likelihood of being victimized. In addition, employee-client contacts were specifically considered in order to measure exposure to potential offenders and assess its impact on violent victimization.

## Research Design & Questions

In the current research, both quantitative and qualitative methods were utilized. Interviews with mental health workers were conducted first, followed by a survey component. Developmentally, the qualitative component was utilized in order to inform the quantitative component. Based on information obtained from interviews, the survey instrument was improved upon. For expansion purposes, the use of both qualitative and quantitative methods added to the current knowledge base by supplying richer information (qualitative component) and increasing generalizability (quantitative component).

As for the research design, Creswell's (1994) "dominant-less dominant design" was employed. "In this design the researcher presents the study within a single, dominant paradigm with one small component of the overall study drawn from the alternative paradigm" (Creswell, 1994, p. 177). In this case, the primary method of data collection involved the use of a questionnaire. In the developmental phase of the questionnaire, qualitative methods were utilized. The purpose of the qualitative component was to pretest the questionnaire, obtain additional information that was used in the final construction of the questionnaire, and collect rich descriptive data that were used to supplement the quantitative findings. In this study, the quantitative portion of the research benefited from qualitative methods being utilized in the survey development phase.

Since violence may be defined differently by various people, involve different actors, occur in different settings, and be reported differently depending on the particular occupation, this study focused on one specific field—mental health. While acts of violence in the workplace may include a number of actors (employees, clients, patients, strangers, etc.), this study focused exclusively on the relationship between employees and clients—specifically mental health clients. Additionally, while violence may occur in various types of workplace situations, this study focused specifically on the violence that occurs within different mental health treatment settings. This includes residential, nonresidential, and crisis settings. To minimize problems related to reporting practices, this study directly surveyed the individual employee in order to determine risk of victimization in the workplace. As noted earlier, victimization surveys indicate that much violence goes unreported altogether. While reporting practices appear different across industries, specifically focusing on one industry—mental health—provides a more complete examination of reporting practices and victimization within this field.

Since there were two components to the research design (qualitative and quantitative), there were separate questions for each component. The qualitative research informed the quantitative research in that feedback was obtained about the survey instrument itself. In addition, the specific qualitative research questions were as follows:

(1) How do mental health professionals define violence in the workplace?

(2) What is the perceived frequency of violence when working with the mentally ill?

(3) Are certain types of mentally ill patients or clients perceived as more prone to violence than others?

(4) When an act of violence occurs, to whom is it generally reported?

(5) What types of precautionary measures may be taken to minimize the threat of violence?

As for the quantitative portion, the following hypotheses were formulated based on a review of the literature. The null hypotheses (Ho) were that there are no significant differences or effects. The first four alternative hypotheses address the concept of potential offenders. Studies have shown that certain types of mentally ill patients or clients are more prone to violence than others (Arango et al., 1999; Link et al., 1992; Modestin & Ammann, 1996; Taylor et al., 1998; Wessely et al., 1994). Higher rates of violence have been associated with more acute mental illness (Modestin & Ammann, 1996). For example, clients having dual diagnoses or schizophrenia have been found to have a greater propensity towards violence than clients with other diagnoses. Therefore, the following hypotheses were explored:

Ha (1): Employees working with the more severe mentally ill are more likely and more often victimized by those clients than employees working with the less severe mentally ill.

Ha (2): Employees who perceive greater danger on the part of their clients are more likely and more often victimized.

In addition, the literature has indicated that the following factors play a role in workplace victimization. They include working with capricious individuals (i.e., health care, social service, or criminal justice settings) and working in crime-prone areas (LaMar et al., 1998; Nigro & Waugh, 1996; NIOSH, 1993a, NIOSH, 1993b; NIOSH, 1996;

Warshaw & Messite, 1996). As such the following hypotheses were explored:

Ha (3):  The greater the number of clients interacted with on a regular basis, the greater the likelihood and frequency of victimization by clients.

Ha (4):  Employees working in urban settings are more likely and more often victimized by clients than those working in rural and suburban settings.

Upon examination of the concept of guardianship, it seems important to consider the environment in which one is employed. According to Warshaw and Messite (1996), "the risk varies with the environment: hospitalized patients, even though they tend to be more severely ill, are perhaps less likely to be violent because of the supervision, care, medication, and support they receive, as compared with those who have been deinstitutionalized and must cope with the stresses of living at home and in the community" (p. 996). Mentally ill clients or patients may pose more of a risk when visiting an outpatient clinic or emergency room, or receiving at-home visits, as compared to being confined at a hospital. Thus, depending on the workplace setting, employees may also be more at risk. As such, this study sought to determine if:

Ha (5):  Employees working in nonresidential and crisis programs are more likely and more often victimized by clients than those working in residential programs.

In addition, the literature has indicated that working solely or in small groups may also play a role in workplace victimization (LaMar et al., 1998; Nigro & Waugh, 1996; NIOSH, 1993a; NIOSH, 1993b; NIOSH, 1996; Warshaw & Messite, 1996). Subsequently, having fewer coworkers present or the absence of capable guardians may play a role in victimization. As such, the following hypothesis was investigated:

Ha (6): The fewer the number of co-workers present while working with clients, the greater the likelihood and frequency of victimization by clients.

Upon examination of the concept of target suitability, the following alternative hypotheses were formulated. According to Nigro and Waugh (1996), trained employees in the area of violence prevention may also make the workplace environment a safer one. As such, the following hypotheses were investigated:

Ha (7): The more violence or crisis prevention training an employee has, the lower the likelihood and frequency of victimization by clients.

Ha (8): The more formal education an employee has, the lower the likelihood and frequency of victimization by clients.

Ha (9): The more job experience an employee has, the lower the likelihood and frequency of victimization by clients.

According to the literature, carrying drugs or having access to drugs and working particular hours or shifts (i.e., late at night or during early morning) have been associated with an increased risk of victimization (LaMar et al., 1998; Nigro & Waugh, 1996; NIOSH, 1993a; NIOSH, 1993b; NIOSH, 1996; Warshaw & Messite, 1996). This suggests the following hypotheses:

Ha (10): Employees who have access to or carry narcotics while working are more likely and more often victimized by clients than those who do not.

Ha (11): Employees working more hours per week and those working late at night or during the early morning are more likely and more often victimized by clients than those who do not.

Last, while demographic characteristics have been found to be statistically significant in victimization research, domain-specific research utilizing routine activities has found that demographic variables (e.g., gender, age) are less significant once routine activities variables are introduced (Lynch, 1987). As such, the following hypothesis was analyzed:

Ha (12):  The routine activities of employees play a greater role in the likelihood and frequency of victimization than do the demographic characteristics of employees.

## Sampling Issues

To conduct this research, a sample of mental health workers was surveyed through the use of a self-administered questionnaire. The unit of analysis was the employee, and the population under study was mental health employees working in Western Pennsylvania. The population, as defined by the Department of Public Welfare-Office of Mental Health under Title 55 of the Pennsylvania Code, was as follows: mental health workers who work in licensed mental health facilities, including outpatient, inpatient, partial hospitalization, crisis, family based, long term structured residence, and community residential rehabilitation. Based on the sampling frame, facilities were limited to those that were licensed, which excluded employees working in private practice. Therefore, generalizations should not be made about individuals who work in private practice, as their clientele or population served may be somewhat different from that of those served by licensed mental health facilities.

The licensed mental health facilities were placed into the following three groups: residential, nonresidential, and crisis. All mental health workers having recurring direct contact with the mentally ill in a treatment capacity were included in the sample. Some examples of such mental health workers include mobile therapists, therapeutic support staff, and counselors. Those who have contact with clients but are not assisting them with a mental health issue were not included in the sample. This includes such workers as those holding administrative, maintenance, or security positions. In addition, visiting psychologists and psychiatrists that are on staff with a treatment facility, but do not have regular contact with clients, were also excluded.

Residential refers to inpatient facilities, long-term structured residence (LTSR), and Community Residential Rehabilitation Services (CRRS), all of which provide living accommodations for clients. Inpatient is defined as a residential treatment setting for diagnosis, evaluation, classification, care and treatment on a continuous 24-hour basis. LTSR is defined as a highly structured therapeutic residential mental health treatment facility serving persons 18 or older who are eligible for hospitalization but who can receive adequate care in a LTSR. A doctor certifies that the patient does not need hospitalization. This may also be a step down for those patients who have previously been hospitalized and may be in transition. CRRS is defined as a transitional program in a community setting for persons with chronic psychiatric disabilities. It provides housing, personal assistance, and psychosocial rehabilitation in a nonmedical setting. There is no time limit, and services are provided to both children and adults.

Nonresidential refers to outpatient facilities, partial hospitalization, and family based services, which do not provide living accommodations for clients. Outpatient facilities are defined as nonresidential treatment settings in which psychiatric, psychological, social, educational and other related services are provided under medical supervision and on a noninpatient basis. Partial hospitalization is defined as a nonresidential treatment modality that includes psychiatric, psychological, social, and vocational elements under medical supervision, provided on a regularly scheduled basis for a minimum of 3 hours per day and less than 24 hours per day. Family based services are in-home programs for children and adolescents under 21 who have a serious mental illness or emotional disturbance and are at risk of psychiatric hospitalization or out of home placement. Services are delivered in a person's residence by a team of two or three mental health professionals.

Crisis refers to telephone services, walk-in services, mobile crisis, medical mobile crisis, and crisis residential, which are provided to clients at the site where they are in crisis. Telephone services refer to 24-hour a day, 7-day-a-week "hotline" services available in each catchment area in Pennsylvania. Calls are screened and referred to the proper crisis counselor. There is one continuous line at all times, no answering machine, no calls put on hold, and no callbacks. Walk-in services are crisis services provided at the provider site. There is face-to-face contact with individuals in crisis or seeking help with persons in crisis. There is no waiting for a crisis counselor. Mobile crisis are services provided at a community site, which is the place where the crisis is occurring or the place where a person in crisis is located. An emergency room or a person's home would be an example of a community site. Medical mobile crisis are services that are provided in the community directly to an individual in crisis and are done by a team consisting of a person authorized to administer medications. For example, a nurse, physician, or nurse practitioner would be authorized to administer medications. Crisis residential services are provided at a small residential facility that has continuous supervision for individuals in crisis. It is a temporary place for someone who needs to be removed from a stressful environment to become stabilized until other arrangements can be made. The maximum stay is 120 hours or 5 days.

In order to obtain a representative sample of mental health workers, stratified cluster sampling was used. Specifically, a one-stage cluster sample was constructed. Cluster sampling was selected, as opposed to other methods, because it was the most efficient way to obtain a probability sample of mental health workers in Western Pennsylvania. The sample was drawn from seven counties in Western Pennsylvania. Since there was not a list in existence of all mental health workers employed in Western Pennsylvania, a list of all licensed mental health facilities was obtained from the Office of Mental Health in Harrisburg, Pennsylvania. Of the seven counties in which the sample was drawn, there are 235 licensed mental health facilities. This list of 235 facilities was stratified into three categories: residential, nonresidential, and crisis. Within each of these categories, there were 56 residential facilities, 159 nonresidential facilities, and 21 crisis facilities.

From this list of facilities, a disproportionate, random sample was drawn, and workers from each of the selected facilities were surveyed for this study. In order to meet the desired sample size, facilities were randomly selected from each category of care until the initial representative sample of employees was produced. Surveys were sent directly to the facility to be distributed to all employees having regular contact with mentally ill clients. Facilities refusing to participate in the study were randomly replaced (only three facilities refused to participate). The final sample size was 449 (a response rate of approximately 37%). As for the total number of employees surveyed within each facility type, 162 worked in nonresidential facilities, 157 worked in residential facilities, and 130 worked in crisis facilities.

As for the qualitative component, interviews (face-to-face and telephone) were conducted for the purposes of pretesting the questionnaire, answering the qualitative research questions, and providing supplemental information to contextualize the quantitative portion. An interview guide was used consisting of general, open-ended questions. The questions are as follows:

(1) In reviewing the survey, are there any questions that are unclear? How would you word them differently?

(2) What do you consider to be violence in the workplace? Do you feel that an occasional violent act is part of the job?

(3) How often have you witnessed violence while working with clients (either to yourself or others)? Do you feel that violence occurs randomly or regularly?

(4) Do you feel that working with certain types of mentally ill patients increases the risk of a violent act occurring? If so, what types?

(5) Do you feel that working in a particular type of setting or environment increases the risk of a violent act occurring? If so, what setting or environment?

(6) What factors do you think contribute to violence in the workplace?

(7) Do you take any precautionary measures while working with clients to prevent violence from occurring? If so, what types of measures?

(8) Have you had violence or crisis prevention training? Do you feel that the training increases one's safety while working? Have you had any other training or education that relates to worker safety? If so, what kinds of training or education?

(9)  Do you feel that worker safety has more to do with education and training or on the job experience or both?

(10) Have you ever reported any violence while working? To whom did you report?

(11) Do you have formal reporting procedures where you work? If so, how did you learn about them? Do you feel that the existence of formal reporting procedures increases the likelihood that one would report a violent act?

For the interviews, purposive and snowball sampling techniques were utilized.  Since nonprobability sampling techniques (purposive and snowball sampling) were used instead of probability sampling techniques, a major limitation was the probable lack of representativeness of the sample.  However, Babbie (1997) states, "occasionally it might be appropriate for you to select your sample on the basis of your own knowledge of the population, its elements, and the nature of your research aims" (p. 97).  Nonprobability sampling techniques were chosen in order to obtain information that was used to gain a better understanding of the problem, answer the research questions, and inform the quantitative portion of the research, but not to make generalizations about the larger population.

Based on the researcher's field contacts, approximately 10 mental health workers, who work in different types of facilities in the seven counties, initially were asked to participate.  If they agreed and did participate, they then were asked if they knew of anyone who might also have knowledge on this subject and would be interested in participating.  The list of referrals was then contacted.

A total of 28 persons were interviewed.  Qualitative methods were employed to the point of redundancy or saturation.  Saturation refers to interviewing to the point where you are confident that little new information will be learned based on what has already been obtained from previous interviews (Rubin & Rubin, 1995).

# Questionnaire

In order to test the hypotheses, a questionnaire was designed to obtain information about employees' routine activities and patterns of criminal victimization. The research design was cross-sectional in nature, which is suitable when the objective is a single-time description.

The questionnaire was administered to examine the relationship between the three central elements of routine activities theory—exposure to potential offenders, guardianship, and target suitability—and victimization at work. Victimization at work was measured as both a dichotomous (yes/no) and continuous (frequency of victimization) dependent variable. In addition, demographic questions pertaining to age, gender, and educational background were asked in order to see if these factors impact on victimization.

In constructing the independent variables, the first concept to be considered was exposure to potential offenders, which is defined as "the visibility of or physical access to victims by potential offenders" (Lynch, 1987, p. 287). The concept of potential offender was substituted for the concept of motivated offender for the reasons noted by Massey et al. (1989). In addition, Bryant and Miller (1997) also noted that a person's actual or perceived risk of victimization is an important indicator in measuring the concept of motivated offender. Thus, to measure this concept, survey items addressed the perceptions of mental health workers regarding the perceived dangerousness of their clients (DANGER), the number of client contacts that employees complete during an average week (CLIENT#), the types of mental illnesses that employees encounter (SCHIZOPHRENIA, SUBSTANCE ABUSE), and the type of community in which they work (RURAL, SUBURBAN, URBAN).

The second concept (guardianship) is defined as "the presence of persons or devices that can prevent or inhibit victimization" (Lynch, 1987, p. 287). To measure this concept, a question asked how many co-workers are typically working nearby during client contacts (#COWORKERS). In addition, a question was asked regarding the type of facility in which the employee works (RESIDENTIAL, NONRESIDENTIAL, CRISIS).

The third concept (target suitability) is defined as "attractiveness as a crime target" (Lynch, 1987, p. 288). To measure this concept, survey items also included questions that asked about previous training in violence or crisis prevention (TRAINING), education (EDUCATION), and number of years experience on the job (EXPERIENCE). In addition, survey items also included demographic questions. Specifically, age (AGE) and gender (GENDER) were included to see how they may or may not relate to the risk of victimization. In addition to these characteristics, a question was also asked pertaining to how the employee relates to clients (STYLE). While this question was based on one's own perception of self in relating with others, it sought to aid in determining if a particular style or manner has any impact on victimization risk. A question was also asked about access to drugs (DRUGS), the number of hours typically worked (HOURS), and the time of day in which one typically worked (DAY).

As for the dependent variable (victimization at work), it is defined as "incidents happening to persons ...while working or on duty" (Lynch, 1987, p. 287). To examine violent victimization, the dependent variable was measured as both a dichotomy and continuous variable. The first question asked respondents whether or not they were ever victims of particular violent acts by their clients. Answers to this question were later used to form three dichotomous dependent variables (VERBAL, THREATS, PHYSICAL). RECENT VERBAL, RECENT THREATS, and RECENT PHYSICAL were formed to examine victimization occurring in the past 12 months, as measured in the second question. Respondents were also asked how many times they were victimized in the past 12 months, which lead to the creation of three continuously measured dependent variables (TOTAL VERBAL, TOTAL THREATS, TOTAL PHYSICAL).

Finally, the following variables were measured in order to provide descriptive information. The survey asked about reporting procedures at the individual facilities (PROCEDURES), whether or not the victim reported their victimization (PRACTICES), and if so, to whom it was reported (SUPERVISOR, COWORKER, POLICE, FRIEND). A question also asked if a weapon was used in the commission of the act (WEAPON). In addition, a question asked mental health workers what they consider to be violence in the workplace (VERBAL ABUSE, THREATS OF HARM, PUSHING, HITTING, KICKING, BITING, PUNCHING, SLAPPING, CHOKING, SPITTING, THROWING OBJECTS, ROBBERY, RAPE, SEXUAL ASSAULT).

# Pretesting Questionnaire & Use of Qualitative Methods

In pretesting the survey, qualitative methods were employed. Pretesting the questionnaire with a purposive sample allowed for the instrument to be fine-tuned (Babbie, 1997). In order to gain detailed information, 23 interviews were conducted one-on-one. In addition, two small groups, consisting of two persons and three persons, were also interviewed. Qualitative interviews allow the researcher to gain an understanding of experiences and events without necessarily participating in those events. The interviewing of respondents was fairly unstructured and primarily done face-to-face. Participants were asked to examine the survey. Questions were posed to respondents regarding their thoughts on the survey. While they did not complete the survey for data collection purposes, they were asked to provide feedback. Short interviews were conducted with the participants to collect additional qualitative data on workplace violence. According to Fowler (1993), interviews are beneficial, especially during the questionnaire development stage.

In selecting participants, it has been suggested that one look for "encultured informants" (Rubin & Rubin, 1995, p. 66). This refers to seeking out persons who have a good understanding of the culture and are able to explain "what it all means." A principle of qualitative sampling is completeness. "You choose people who are knowledgeable about the subject and talk with them until what you hear provides an overall sense of meaning of a concept, theme, or process" (Rubin & Rubin, 1995, p. 73). Therefore, both purposeful and snowball sampling techniques were employed.

Maxwell (1996) defines purposeful sampling as "a strategy in which particular settings, persons, or events are selected deliberately in order to provide important information that can not be obtained well from other sources" (p. 70). Initially, participants were known to the researcher and sought out because of their experience in the field of mental health and the type of information they could provide. Subsequently, those participants were asked if they knew of any other knowledgeable persons who may want to participate, and those referrals were contacted (snowball sampling). Again, interviews were conducted until no new information was learned. Every effort was made to ensure that there was diversity among the respondents. Interviews were conducted at various locations. Permission was sought from either the director or manager to conduct an interview within a particular.

During the interview process, notes were taken, and the interviews recorded via a tape recorder, with the participants' permission. While recording interviews allows for greater accuracy in the information obtained, there are some disadvantages. According to Rubin and Rubin (1995), a tape recorder may give the appearance of formality in situations that are generally set up to be informal. It may result in participants holding back information. Also, recording interviews requires attention. For example, one needs to make sure that the batteries work or the sound quality is adequate. Even if one is using a recorder, it is recommended that notes still be taken as a backup in case there is a problem with the recording of the interviews. Finally, in honoring the participants' right to confidentiality, no identifying information was included in the transcripts. Furthermore, respondents were strongly advised not to use any identifying information during the interviews. This included both employee and institutional identifiers.

## Administration of Survey

All facilities selected were contacted both in writing and in person or by phone in order to request their participation in this study. Once access was granted, all mental health workers that fit the criteria were invited to participate. The self-administered questionnaire was mailed (or hand delivered) to all participants at their place of employment, to be distributed by the designated person (management or human resources). Surveys were either distributed to employees via their mailboxes or were included along with their paychecks. Utilizing a similar distribution strategy, response rates have varied, with a minimum response rate averaging 30% (Harris & Benson, 1998). In order to increase the response rate, personal visits to the facilities were made wherever possible.

All participants were notified via a cover letter that their participation in the survey research was voluntary, and that they would be guaranteed complete anonymity. The cover letter also provided a brief discussion of why the research was being conducted. A stamped, self-addressed envelope was enclosed for participants to return the survey. Returned questionnaires provided evidence of implied consent.

In order to increase the response rate, several steps were taken. First, if possible, arrangements to meet directly with management or to attend staff meetings were made in order to introduce the research project and briefly discuss the importance of the survey. At this point, surveys were distributed. In addition, it was also made clear in the cover letter that all surveys would be returned directly to the researcher to minimize risk to employees and to guard against coercion. Management would not be aware of participants' individual survey information or their participation in general. Furthermore, a letter was mailed to all participating facilities outlining the desired distribution method and the importance of voluntary participation. Last, a follow up mailing was conducted approximately one week after the initial surveys were distributed. The same number of letters was delivered as was used for the surveys. The follow-up letter was distributed to the same sampled facilities encouraging their participation in the survey and stating the researcher's appreciation.

## Human Subjects Issues

The human subjects issues that needed to be addressed were anonymity and confidentiality, no harm to participants, deception, voluntary participation, and informed consent (Babbie, 1995). First, all participants' answers were kept confidential for the qualitative component. While the researcher may be able to identify a particular response with a respondent, the data were ultimately presented in aggregate form that ensures confidentially. In other words, a particular response would not be identifiable to a particular respondent in the finished product. In addition, all employee and institutional identifiers were deleted from the transcriptions. Informed consent forms were given to all participants in the qualitative component that outlined the issue of confidentiality.

As for the quantitative data, in order to maintain anonymity, respondents were instructed not to put any identifying information on the survey, which was outlined in the cover letter. In addition, there would be no way for employers to determine who participated in the research, as management would not be administering the surveys. This was also addressed in the cover letter, as well as in a letter addressed to all facilities that agree to participate.

Second, no matter what type of research is conducted, there is always the chance that someone may be injured or harmed (Babbie, 1995). In this case, there was the chance that a participant would become uncomfortable with the research topic, especially if they had been victimized. To minimize any negative feelings, participants were given a brief overview of the research project in the cover letter and the informed consent form. Subsequently, participants were made aware that the questionnaire was specifically designed to measure victimization at work and that the survey asked about the respondent's own personal experiences. Respondents participating in the qualitative component of the research were informed that their responses would be utilized to revise the survey, as well as provide descriptive information about victimization in the workplace. They were also advised that the questions would ask about victimization, as well as their own personal experience. All participants were advised that should they feel uncomfortable with the subject matter, they should not feel obligated to participate. This was also outlined in the cover letter and the informed consent form. Participants were instructed that their participation was completely voluntary and that they could stop participating in the research project at any time. No deception was used at any point in the research process.

The last issue concerns voluntary participation and informed consent. All respondents participating in the survey did so voluntarily. They were informed of what the research process entailed via the cover letter and informed consent form. In addition, they were also advised that the research was independent of their employment. As stated before, all participants were made aware of the general purpose of the study, informed of any risks, and were made aware that they may withdraw from the process at any time. Again, the process was outlined to all participants in both the cover letter and informed consent form. A copy of the informed consent form was given to all participants interviewed, and the researcher also retained a copy. The return of the questionnaire provided evidence of implied consent.

# CHAPTER IV

# The Practitioner's Perspective

The interviews conducted with the mental health workers provided descriptive data that informed and complemented the quantitative data, and allowed for an opportunity to fine-tune the survey instrument. The survey instrument was given to each interviewee for the purpose of gathering feedback about the clarity of the questions. The purpose of reviewing the survey was not to collect survey data from the interviewees, but rather the survey was revised based on the information received from the participants. Twenty-eight persons employed in mental health were interviewed across seven counties. Twenty-three individual interviews were conducted and the other five participants were interviewed in small groups. Eight of those interviewed worked in a residential setting, eight worked in a nonresidential setting, and seven worked in a crisis setting.

## Defining Violence in the Workplace

When defining violence in the workplace, one could say that there is a spectrum of violence. At one end of the spectrum, there are acts of verbal abuse and threats; and, at the other end, there are physical acts of violence. Overall, there is a wide range of behaviors occurring in between the two ends of the spectrum. What one employee considers violence, someone else may define as part of the job or simply an annoyance. For example, some interviewees considered verbal threats to be violence. One employee working in a nonresidential setting said, "Workplace violence is feeling threatened or being physically threatened, as well as being verbally abused." A crisis worker characterized the start of workplace violence as "a verbal escalation that creates a stressful environment." Another crisis worker stated, "Workplace violence is any form of behavior that could be construed at any level as dangerous." Finally, an employee working in a nonresidential setting said, "Verbal assaults can be just as frightening across the board to all involved."

Continuing through the spectrum, some interviewees believed that violence was more than just swearing or verbal abuse alone. For example, some interviewees experienced swearing or verbal abuse all the time and considered it part of the job. One employee working in a residential setting said, "There are degrees of violence, and profanity alone would not be considered violence....Verbal threats, I would consider violence." Verbal threats appeared to be the next level in the spectrum and were taken seriously by many of those interviewed, especially when a weapon or object was involved. A crisis worker said, "Workplace violence means verbal threats with a means of carrying out threats." An employee working in a nonresidential setting stated, "It (workplace violence) is more than verbal, but rather physical threats of assault." Finally, another employee working in a nonresidential setting said, "There is some verbal, but I consider workplace violence to be more physical."

It should be noted that differences in how employees defined workplace violence did not appear to depend upon the location or type of facility in which one worked. However, while not everyone considered acts such as verbal abuse, swearing, or threats of physical harm to be violence, all interviewees unanimously defined violence to include physical acts. Physical acts may include behaviors such as pushing, hitting, kicking, biting, punching, slapping, choking, spitting, throwing objects, robbery, rape, and other types of sexual assault. Physical acts of violence may be carried out using weapons, objects, fists, or another part of the body. One employee working in a nonresidential setting said, "Workplace violence is any act of aggression that has the potential of causing physical harm or extreme mental anguish to any person involved in the incident." Another employee working in a nonresidential setting stated, "Workplace violence is an act that results in bodily harm, and it is not threats, swearing, or verbal abuse."

# Perceived Frequency of Violence

While definitions of workplace violence varied, many interviewees had experienced workplace violence on some level and considered it part of the job. As for their perceptions of danger, they seemed to vary. While nearly all of those interviewed could remember an incident of violence, most believed that they were not in any real danger. One employee working in a nonresidential setting said, "The potential for violence is always present, and it is something you have to constantly monitor, be aware of, and not take for granted." In working with this population, a crisis worker stated, "You need to be prepared for it (violence)."

Many of the interviewees said that there is a chance that one may be confronted with a violent person or someone who has violent tendencies. Again, this was attributed to the population that employees have contact with on a regular basis. One employee working in a residential setting said, "If they (patient, client, or consumer) become unstable, there is a potential for violence." Throughout the interviews, the terms patient, client, and consumer were used interchangeably. All three terms are considered appropriate in the field.

Another employee working in a residential setting stated, "We deal with a lot of anger and anxiety in working with folks with mental health problems....Violence is rare, but workers need to be prepared for it and need to handle it." Finally, an employee working in a nonresidential setting said, "I feel pretty lucky, as there is always the possibility of violence, but I do not think and worry about it."

Overall, most of the interviewees characterized violence as occurring on a sporadic basis. Again, it did not seem to make a difference whether the employee worked in a residential, nonresidential, or crisis setting. Physical acts of violence were considered to occur infrequently. Furthermore, many believed that violence did not just come out of the blue, but rather, indicators or warning signs were generally evident.

While most of the employees interviewed stated that violence did not occur on a regular basis, some interviewees characterized verbal abuse and swearing as occurring on a more frequent basis. Thus, if violence was unanimously defined to include verbal acts, then violence in the workplace would be occurring more often. However, many of those interviewed did not include profanity or verbal abuse in their definition of violence.  Rather, verbal acts appeared to be more commonplace and generally thought of as part of the job when dealing with this population.  Verbal acts were not necessarily construed as violence and not viewed in the same manner as physical acts.  As stated previously, physical acts were considered to occur infrequently.

Overall, most of the interviewees conveyed the message that violence in this field is not as frequent as people think, which is consistent with previous literature (Bower, 1998; Monahan & Arnold, 1996; Steadman et al., 1998).  However, it does appear that there is some controversy or inconsistency regarding the frequency of violence, which has been the case in previous literature as well (Baron & Neuman, 1996; Capozzoli & McVey, 1996; Labig, 1995; Monahan & Arnold, 1996; Nigro & Waugh, 1996; Warshaw & Messite, 1996).  It would seem, then, that the perceived frequency of violence in this field depends upon how violence is defined, and what experiences are viewed as simply part of the job.

## Perceptions Towards the Mentally Ill

The general consensus among those interviewed was that the mentally ill are no more violent than anyone else in the general population. Many attributed the stereotypes given to the mentally ill as growing out of fear and the media.  These perceptions are consistent with some of the literature that addresses the mental illness-violence connection (Bower, 1998; Martel & Dietz, 1992; Monahan & Arnold, 1996; Steadman et al., 1998).  One employee working in a nonresidential setting said, "Violence is part of the job because you are dealing with people in general and it is inherent in society, not just the mentally ill." Another stated, "When working with the public, you get an increased risk of violence."

Most of those interviewed were not quick to say that particular diagnoses were more prone to violence than others.  One employee working in a nonresidential setting said, "The ones we least expect are the ones that follow through (carry out violence)....I don't feel that there is enough information to make that determination."  Rather, when examining proneness to violence, it may be necessary to look at other factors that are coming into play that exacerbate the illness.

For example, clients who are decompensating or very symptomatic may be at an increased risk for violence. One employee working in a residential setting said, "Any type of mentally ill client, if unstable, can become violent....If decompensating, get them help." Another stated, "Risk is not diagnoses based, but rather we need to look at the whole picture of the consumer." For example, clients who have no social support, a prior abuse history, and substance abuse issues may be at an increased risk. One employee working in a nonresidential setting said, "If violence is a way of life for them, it is their behavior pattern and normal for them...Violence is how it is settled...A norm within the community." Other interviewees working in residential settings believed that working with those in the criminally insane or forensic populations were also more prone to violence.

Another factor that played a role in one's perception of propensity towards violence was use of medications. Many of those interviewed indicated that if a client was using his or her medications properly, there was generally not an increased risk towards violence. However, for clients who either went off their medications completely or had adjustment problems, employee perceptions were that an increased risk of violence was possible. One employee who worked in a nonresidential setting said, "When on medications, consumers are usually fine and operate in society very well....When consumers go off medications you will see odd behavior and they act out of character." This is consistent with the literature that found that those who failed to take prescribed medications were more likely to be violent (Bartels et al., 1991; Kasper et al., 1997; Martell & Dietz, 1992; Smith, 1989; Swartz et al., 1998; Taylor, 1985).

While most interviewees believed that other factors needed to be examined in addition to the specific diagnoses, the following diagnoses were believed to be most associated with an increased risk of violence. About half of the interviewees associated schizophrenia and other psychotic disorders with an increased risk of violence. This is also consistent with the literature that states schizophrenic patients have an increased risk of offending (Arango et al., 1999; Link et al., 1992; Modestin & Ammann, 1996; Taylor et al., 1998; Wessely et al., 1994). Approximately 25% associated borderline and other personality disorders with an increased risk of violence. About one-third of those interviewed believed that there was an increased risk of violence among those with substance-related disorders. In most cases, interviewees believed that the risk was higher among those clients with comorbidity or a dual diagnosis. This is also consistent with the literature that states having both a mental illness and a substance abuse problem results in a greater propensity towards violence (Bartels et al., 1991; Swanson et al., 1990). Other diagnoses mentioned less frequently included bipolar and other mood disorders, impulse-control disorders, and childhood disorders.

In addition to specific diagnoses, perceptions of an increased risk of violence among patients were also based on the type of services the patient was receiving. For example, some interviewees believed that consumers who were currently in a residential or inpatient setting were more likely to act out than consumers in other types of settings. Those interviewed attributed this to the fact that consumers in residential and inpatient settings are generally sicker and more unstable than those who are living in the community, which is why they are receiving more intensive services. In addition, mental health workers spend more time with clients in residential and inpatient settings, which may allow more opportunities for violence to occur.

On the other hand, some interviewees believed that working with clients in the community, in crisis situations, could also pose a risk. This may be due to the fact that when consumers are in crisis, generally they are unstable and decompensating, which may increase their propensity towards violence. One crisis worker said, "When a consumer is in a crisis state, they are much more volatile....You also see heightened symptomology." There is also less structure when they are living in the community, which can be an added stressor when the consumer is in crisis. In addition, if clients are in crisis and are involuntarily committed, this may also pose an increased risk of violence. Another crisis worker said, "When clients are threatened with loss of freedom or a perceived loss, they sometimes react." Bringing a consumer to the emergency room when in a crisis state may also increase the risk of violence. One employee working in a nonresidential setting stated, "The intensity level is high in the emergency room environment, and typically emergency rooms don't like psychiatric patients because they are difficult and take a lot of time....They can be combative and loud." This is consistent with the literature that states hospital emergency rooms have been witnessing increased violence by former clients and patients (Carroll, 1996; Hoag-Apel, 1998; Sullivan & Yuan, 1995; Warshaw & Messite, 1996).

Another setting where clients were viewed to possibly pose an increased risk included outpatient settings, especially involving those services that included home visits. One employee working in a nonresidential setting said, "You may be at an increased risk when providing mobile therapy, because you are in the consumer's home and it is more difficult to control the environment....Certainly, any setting where all the precautions you would like to take can not be taken increases your risk." In other cases, employees reported that clients might also pose an increased risk if the services (home visits) are mandated by the court and not wanted by the consumer. This is also consistent with the literature that states clients having to deal with stressors in the community may pose a greater risk because they are receiving less structured services as compared to hospitalized patients (Warshaw & Messite, 1996).

## Reporting Violence

Most of the interviewees had reported an act of violence at some point in their career. Some of the reporting was done in the capacity as the immediate supervisor, and some of the reporting was done as the victim. Most of the interviewees had formal reporting procedures in place where they worked, and thus were educated about these procedures through orientation (covered in the policy/procedure manual), in-service trainings, and on-the-job experience.

In general, the reporting of such acts was done internally. The immediate supervisor was generally notified first. Other personnel who also worked with the client would also be notified so that everyone would be kept up to date. The severity of the incident would determine the types of reports to be filed. For example, all of the interviewees stressed the need for documentation. In some cases, documentation would take the form of an internal incident report. This report would stay within the immediate facility and the incident would also be documented in the client's file. However, if the incident was determined to be serious, a report would also be filed with the county Mental Health/Mental Retardation (MH/MR) and the regional offices. In this case, an unusual incident report would be filed with these offices. According to one employee working in a residential setting, "Internally documented incidents are not always put in the form of an unusual incident report, but all unusual incident reports are documented internally."

Depending on the seriousness of the situation, 911 may be called. Most of the interviewees indicated that the police were not involved unless some type of physical act resulting in bodily harm or medical treatment had occurred, or if charges were to be filed. One crisis worker said, "I discussed the threat with my supervisor instead of the police, because the threat was not taken seriously." Another employee working in a nonresidential setting said, "Calling the police depends on the acuteness of the situation." These reporting practices are consistent with the literature. Overall, there appear to be differences in reporting practices for certain industries (Peek-Asa et al., 1998; Warchol, 1998). Typically, the mental health field experiences more victimization than is shown by police reports. This is due to reporting practices among this field whereby employees would report the violent act directly to their employer, as opposed to reporting it to the police. In other cases, the act may not be reported to the police, or even to the employer for that matter, because it is not recognized as workplace violence (NIOSH, 1996, Warshaw & Messite, 1996). This is consistent with interviewee statements that they would only report to the police if it were a serious incident or the situation warranted calling the police. Again, reporting to the police appears to be based on perceptions of the individual worker as to how they view the situation. There do not appear to be any hard and fast rules.

Overall, the interviewees who had experienced some type of violence did report the act to their employer and other officials (if viewed as necessary). Most believed that having formal procedures in place increased the likelihood of reporting. One employee working in a residential setting stated, "Reporting is mandatory and is used because the supervisor follows up." Another interviewee said, "Everything is documented....There is a staff log, a medication log, and a communication log....We document all actions of consumers and ourselves (employee)." Documentation was stressed among many of those interviewed. For example, one employee working in a nonresidential setting stated, "Document, document, document, report, report, report...Incidents are reported because it is drilled into your head." In most cases, formal procedures were in place and the staff was trained regarding those procedures. One employee working in a nonresidential setting said, "There are formal procedures at all levels—state, county, and agency levels....The procedures give you steps on how to complete unusual incident reports, log notes, daily activities, case notes....Everything is filed and documented....It is part of what you do." One crisis worker stated, "Making employees aware during orientation about policies and procedures increases reporting because they know about it and if in doubt they ask....Communication is the big thing." Some interviewees also believed that by not reporting, you would be doing yourself and your agency a disservice. For example, one employee working in a residential setting said, "I would probably report regardless of formal procedures....Nip this stuff in the bud....If you let it go, it will build....If you don't do something, it affects other patients and leads to chaos."

While all of the interviewees experiencing some type of violence had gone through the reporting procedures, some believed that there still might be some staff that does not report. One employee working in a nonresidential setting said, "I think there is a lot of nonreporting among staff....They may not report because they are not thinking about it, or fear having some incrimination legally, or the possibility of a lawsuit, or they may fear losing their funding if they have a lot of reports." Another interviewee said, "I do not think that having formal procedures increases reporting among staff....They may not report because of embarrassment and don't want to be caught making that kind of error." In addition to personal liability, some of the interviewees believed that staff would not report for other reasons. For example, one employee working in a nonresidential setting stated, "Some people (staff) may not report if nothing happened (an injury did not occur) as to avoid filling out paperwork." Another employee working in a residential setting said, "Some staff don't report because they have too much empathy....They don't report because they don't want to get the consumer in trouble."

## Precautionary Measures

In addition to trainings on formal procedures regarding reporting incidences, employees are also trained on how to protect themselves, and some agencies required other safety measures to be taken. Such precautionary measures may be included in the policy/procedure manual and discussed at orientation, be included within in-service trainings, or be learned through on-the-job experiences. The types of precautionary measures used by the interviewees and agencies varied. For example, it was reported that one nonresidential agency had procedures that included an established verbal alarm that, when spoken aloud, would indicate to other staff that there was a problem. For instance, "I need to see Al" would be the code for help. The agency also had panic buttons and maintained general security on site. Another employee working in a nonresidential setting said, "Our agency has a phone that we just pick up which is a direct line to the police." Another interviewee said that their agency (residential) had signs posted that read "No Firearms" and required staff to wear ID badges and clients to check in with the receptionist. Other reported safety precautions maintained at agencies included keeping all medications under lock and key, having locked security doors (limiting access to clients), having a policy in place regarding contacting police, and using intercom systems and metal detectors. All of those interviewed stated that their agency took some type of precautionary measures, whether it was in a residential, nonresidential, or crisis setting.

In addition to safety measures taken by agencies, interviewees discussed many precautions that could be taken by employees on their own accord. For example, the physical layout of the room could increase perceptions of safety. Interviewees suggested that the room be set up so that employees are closest to the door. Also, attempts may be made to maintain a reasonable distance between employees and the consumer. In addition, workers can ensure that there are no sharp objects within the consumer's reach, on a desk or in the room. Also, before the consumer arrives for an appointment, employees may decide whether or not to close the door, and if they should have other staff present. One employee working in a nonresidential setting said, "Depending on the person, I will consider whether or not other people need to be around." Increasing the number of staff present may also increase safety as well. Other interviewees suggested that maintaining appropriate boundaries is necessary, as well as not giving out personal information (i.e., home telephone number, address, etc.). One crisis worker said, "Be aware of what is going on around you....Stay calm in your approach with clients." Sometimes body language or tone of voice may be enough to set off a client.

Most interviewees said that their agencies provided training in the area of safety. The most common training mentioned was crisis prevention and intervention training. This training focuses on the use of passive physical restraints, physical maneuverings, verbal de-escalation, and self-defense. Basically, the training teaches what to do in a crisis situation. One employee working in a residential setting said, "Crisis prevention intervention training is helpful....It teaches you protection and ways to keep yourself safe and not harm anyone else."

In addition, first aid training was also common. Trainings such as these address how to handle clients that used needles, taking safety precautions (such as wearing rubber gloves), and how to dispose of hazardous waste. Overall, training appeared to be one area that aided in maintaining safety. One employee working in a nonresidential setting said, "Training gives you more confidence that you could protect yourself." Another employee said, "Continual training is necessary....It is that skill that you don't always have to use, that you need to keep current in case you have to use it."

While most of the interviewees believed that trainings were helpful, many also maintained that ensuring safety had more to do with a combination of experience and training. Some suggested that keeping safe had more to do with common sense. Others believed that while they learned some safety techniques from training, most of what they learned was from experience or by talking with others in the field. One crisis worker said, "You can have trainings, but until you are put in a situation that you have to use it, you don't know what you will do." Another employee working in a nonresidential setting said, "Training can be effective, but you also need to have the experience yourself."

However, despite the value of experience, not everyone has the opportunity to gain the necessary experience. One employee working in a nonresidential setting said, "Experience is by far the best and seeing your techniques working....Fortunately, we don't have enough situations for staff to get the experience, so trainings are necessary." Another employee working in a residential setting stated, "Training gives those fresh out of school a chance to give them skills to keep them safe." Finally, others believed that trainings forced them to pay attention and consider different situations that might not otherwise have received any thought. One employee working in a residential setting said, "At a minimum, training increases one's awareness." Another employee working in a nonresidential setting stated, "Training is important, because training increases awareness....Experience alone gets you too comfortable, and you assume nothing is going to happen." Overall, many of those interviewed learned how to increase their safety through on-the-job experience. However, most believed that trainings in conjunction with experience were important in maintaining safety. Finally, one employee working in a nonresidential setting said, "Training is important in order to educate employees on how to protect themselves, not experience...When we first started, we didn't have any job experience."

## Summary

Based on the interviews, there appeared to be a general consensus of what is considered violence in the workplace. While some did not consider profanity or verbal abuse to be violence, all considered physical acts to be violence. As for the likelihood of violence occurring in the workplace, most had experienced some type of violence in one form or another. However, most did not consider their job to be particularly dangerous, nor did they consider violence to be a regular occurrence. Most believed that any acts of violence were sporadic and infrequent. With the exception of profanity or verbal abuse, most believed that violence in this field is not as common as people believe.

As for their perceptions about the mentally ill, all of those interviewed stated that the mentally ill are no more violent than anyone else in the general population. This attitude is also consistent with the literature (Bower, 1998; Monahan & Arnold, 1996; Steadman et al., 1998). Most of the interviewees did not believe that a particular diagnosis alone would be associated with an increased risk of violence, but rather believed that other factors may in fact exacerbate the illness. For example, medication issues, family issues, the symptomology of the illness, and their living situation (i.e., residential, inpatient, reside in community) were just a few of the factors that were noted. While most contended that it was important to examine other factors, schizophrenia and other psychotic disorders, borderline and other personality disorders, and substance-related disorders were the three most common diagnoses where increased risks of violence were seen in patients. This is also consistent with the literature, as schizophrenia and substance-related disorders have been cited as contributing to a greater propensity towards violence, as compared to other disorders (Bartels et al., 1991; Kasper et al., 1997; Martell & Dietz, 1992; Smith, 1989; Swartz et al., 1998; Taylor, 1985).

When violence does occur, all of those interviewed stated that it was reported in one form or another. Most of the interviewees had reported an act of violence at some point in their career. Formal reporting procedures were common and generally introduced at orientation, and the importance of reporting was reaffirmed through continual in-service trainings. In most cases, the reporting was done internally. However, outside agencies (i.e., county and regional Mental Health/Mental Retardation offices, police) would be notified if the incident were deemed of a serious nature. What would be considered serious appeared to vary among interviewees. This is also consistent with the literature, in that this field has generally shown higher rates of victimization in victimization surveys as compared to what is suggested by police reports (Peek-Asa et al., 1998; Warchol, 1998). While those interviewed generally reported the incident, some believed that there was some underreporting among staff. They believed that this was due to fear of liability, not wanting to get the client in trouble, and either not wanting or forgetting to fill out the paperwork.

Overall, none of the interviewees believed that their job was extremely dangerous. Most stated that their agencies had taken precautionary measures in the workplace designed to keep employees safe. In addition, there were many other safety measures that employees could take to further ensure their safety when working with clients. Some of the safety measures were introduced at orientation, while others were learned through trainings and on-the-job experience. While some believed that experience played a greater role in keeping them safe, most believed that it was more of a combination of experience and training.

Based on the qualitative results, it appears that the perceived frequency of violence is low when working with the mentally ill. As such, the expected findings from the quantitative data should be similar. In addition, while some of the qualitative data suggested that patients afflicted with schizophrenia and substance-related disorders might be more prone to violence, other contributing factors were noted as well. When an act of violence does occur, it is most often reported internally. It is therefore expected that the quantitative findings will also show that most acts of violence are reported to the employer rather than the police. Finally, the qualitative data showed that both facilities and individual employees took precautionary measures. Education, training, and on-the-job experience were put forth as useful in preventing violence. Therefore, it is expected that the quantitative findings will also reflect lesser victimization among those employees with greater education, training, and experience. The next chapter addresses the quantitative results of this study.

# CHAPTER V

# Violence in Mental Health

In this chapter, the results from the statistical analyses are discussed. The descriptive statistics are presented first, followed by the multivariate results. Both logistic and linear regression models are presented. Discussion of the models takes place based on three different types of victimization: verbal abuse, threats of violence, and physical acts of violence. Consideration of the individual hypotheses also follows.

## Descriptive Statistics

The first seven independent variables were used in measuring exposure to potential offenders. The descriptive statistics for these variables are presented in Table 1. The first variable to be discussed is DANGER. The respondents were asked how many of their client contacts per week were dangerous to their person. The range of answers varied from zero to 60 and was coded accordingly. The mean was 2.84, indicating that the average employee viewed approximately three of their weekly client contacts as dangerous. Interestingly enough, over half of those surveyed indicated that they believed that none or only one of their weekly client contacts posed a threat of danger. Approximately 80% of those surveyed indicated that they believed that three or less of their weekly client contacts were dangerous, and 90% believed that six or less of their weekly client contacts posed a danger. Due to the impact that outliers have on the mean, one case was removed in order to

*Workplace Violence and Mental Illness*

examine its impact on the mean. In this case, when the outlier was removed, the mean decreased slightly from 2.84 to 2.71.

Table 1—Descriptive Statistics—Exposure To Potential Offenders

| Variable | Mean | SD | N |
|---|---|---|---|
| DANGER | 2.84 | 5.87 | 436 |
| CLIENT# | 25.41 | 27.22 | 440 |
| SCHIZOPHRENIA | 0.60 | 0.49 | 448 |
| SUBSTANCE ABUSE | 0.37 | 0.48 | 448 |
| RURAL | 0.24 | 0.43 | 433 |
| SUBURBAN | 0.35 | 0.48 | 433 |
| URBAN | 0.41 | 0.49 | 433 |

The next variable, CLIENT#, refers to the total number of face-to-face client contacts an employee had on a weekly basis. The number of client contacts on a weekly basis ranged from zero to 240. The mean was 25.41, which indicates that the average worker had 25 client contacts on a weekly basis. As with the DANGER variable, CLIENT# also had a case that was an outlier. As with the DANGER variable, the outlier was removed, and the mean decreased from 25.41 to 24.92.

The next two variables refer to types of mental illnesses (i.e., SCHIZOPHRENIA and SUBSTANCE ABUSE). Respondents were asked to check the top three types of mental illnesses that they deal with most often. Based on the literature, schizophrenia and substance abuse were selected as the variables of interest, and both were then coded as either zero or one. For both variables, zero meant that the employee did not often deal with schizophrenics or substance abusers, and one meant that the employee did often deal with schizophrenics or substance abusers. The mean for SCHIZOPHRENIA was .60, indicating that 60% of the respondents reported working regularly with schizophrenics. The mean for SUBSTANCE ABUSE was .37, indicating that 37% worked regularly with clients with substance-related problems.

The last three variables examined relate to the type of community in which respondents reported working (RURAL, SUBURBAN, and URBAN). The variables were coded as either a zero or a one for all three variables. For example, for the variable RURAL, zero meant that the employee did not work in a rural environment, and one meant that the employee did work in a rural environment. The mean score for RURAL was .24, indicating that 24% of the respondents worked in a rural area. The mean score for SUBURBAN was .35, which means that 35% of those surveyed were employed in a suburban area. The mean score for URBAN was .41, indicating that 41% of the employees worked in an urban area.

The next four independent variables were used in order to measure the concept of guardianship. The descriptive statistics for these variables are presented in Table 2. The first variable refers to the typical number of coworkers present while one is working with clients (# COWORKERS). The answers varied from zero to 150. The mean score was 5.18, indicating that the average number of coworkers present during client contacts was five. Approximately 25% of the respondents reported typically working alone. As stated previously, because of the impact that outliers have on the mean, one case was removed to examine its impact. In this case, the mean decreased from 5.18 to 4.85.

Table 2—Descriptive Statistics—Guardianship

| Variable | Mean | SD | N |
|----------|------|------|-----|
| #COWORKERS | 5.18 | 13.06 | 438 |
| NONRESIDENTIAL | 0.36 | 0.48 | 449 |
| RESIDENTIAL | 0.35 | 0.48 | 449 |
| CRISIS | 0.29 | 0.45 | 449 |

The next three variables refer to the type of facility in which one works (NONRESIDENTIAL, RESIDENTIAL, and CRISIS). Outpatient, partial hospitalization, and family based services were considered NONRESIDENTIAL. Inpatient, community residential rehabilitation, and long-term structured residence were considered RESIDENTIAL. Crisis facilities were labeled CRISIS. The variables were coded in the same manner as for type of community, which was zero and one. The mean score for NONRESIDENTIAL was .36, indicating that 36% of those surveyed worked in a nonresidential facility. The mean score for RESIDENTIAL was .35, which shows that 35% of those surveyed worked in residential facilities. The mean score for CRISIS was .29, indicating that 29% of the respondents reported working in a crisis facility.

The last nine independent variables were used as measures for the concept of target suitability. The descriptive statistics for these variables are presented in Table 3. The first variable refers to the number of hours of violence or crisis prevention training the employee had during the past year (TRAINING). The variable was coded as a continuous variable, with a range of zero to 200. The mean score was 6.46, indicating that the average amount of violence or crisis prevention training employees experienced in the past year was 6 _ hours. As with a few other independent variables, one outlier was removed, and the mean decreased from 6.46 to 6.02.

The next variable refers to the education level of the employee (EDUCATION). The variable was coded as follows: some high school (0), GED or high school diploma (1), some college or post-secondary schooling (2), Associate Degree (3), Bachelor Degree (4), some graduate work (5), or a graduate degree (6). The range was one to six, indicating that all respondents had a minimum of a GED or high school diploma. The mean was 4.36, indicating that the average employee had a Bachelor degree. In fact, one-third of the respondents had a bachelor degree and another third had a graduate degree.

The next variable refers to the number of years of experience the respondent had in the field of mental health (EXPERIENCE). The variable was coded as a continuous variable, with a range of one month to 39 years of experience. The mean score was 9.08, indicating that the average worker had approximately nine years experience in mental health.

The next variable refers to the age of the respondent (AGE). This variable was also coded as a continuous variable, with a range of 18 to 69 years. The mean score was 39.46, which shows that the average employee was approximately 39 1/2 years old.

Table 3—Descriptive Statistics—Target Suitability

| Variable | Mean | SD | N |
|----------|------|------|-----|
| TRAINING | 6.46 | 13.91 | 445 |
| EDUCATION | 4.36 | 1.51 | 447 |
| EXPERIENCE | 9.08 | 7.66 | 441 |
| AGE | 39.46 | 11.54 | 444 |
| GENDER | 0.73 | 0.44 | 447 |
| STYLE | 5.14 | 3.81 | 447 |
| DRUGS | 0.37 | 0.48 | 443 |
| HOURS | 38.97 | 8.29 | 447 |
| DAY | 0.63 | 0.48 | 446 |

The next variable refers to the sex of the respondent (GENDER). Males were coded as a zero, and females were coded as a one. The mean score was .73, indicating that 73% of those surveyed were female.

The next variable to be discussed refers to the self-reported style or demeanor of the employee while working with clients (STYLE). The respondents were asked to characterize their style on a scale of zero to ten (i.e., 0=very relaxed/laid back; 10=very assertive/firm). The mean score was 5.14, indicating that the average employee was in the middle of the two ends of the spectrum.

The next variable refers to whether or not the employee had access to or carried drugs while working (DRUGS). The variable was coded as either a zero or a one. If the employee did not have any access to drugs, the variable was coded as a zero. If the employee had access to drugs, the variable was coded as a one. The mean score was .37, indicating that 37% of those surveyed had access to or carried drugs while working.

The next variable refers to the average number of hours the employee worked per week (HOURS). The variable was coded continuously, with a range of six to 80 hours per week. The mean score was 38.97, which shows that the average employee worked almost 39 hours per week. Again, the presence of an outlier warranted a comparison between the means once the outlier had been removed. In this case, the mean only decreased slightly from 38.97 to 38.88.

The last independent variable to be discussed refers to the time of day in which the employee reported working on a regular basis (DAY). The variable was coded as either a zero or a one. If the employee did not typically work during the day, it was coded as a zero. If the employee did typically work during the day, it was coded as a one. The mean score was .63, indicating that 63% of those surveyed reported typically working during the day.

The survey asked respondents two questions regarding victimization. The first question asked whether or not they had ever been a victim of any of the following by a client: verbal abuse or swearing, threats of physical harm, pushing, hitting, kicking, biting, punching, slapping, choking, spitting, throwing objects, robbery, rape, and other types of sexual assault. The second question asked respondents how many times in the past 12 months they had experienced any of those acts. The data from these two questions were utilized in the following manner in order to create nine separate dependent variables.

First, victimization was separated into the following three categories: verbal abuse, threats of physical harm, and physical acts of violence. Thus, the data for verbal abuse and threats were obtained directly from the two survey questions that asked about verbal abuse and threats. For physical acts of violence, the data were combined from the rest of the categories, which included pushing, hitting, kicking, biting, punching, slapping, choking, spitting, throwing objects, robbery, rape, and other types of sexual assault. All of these acts were combined and put into one category because there was relatively little victimization reported for each type of the physical acts.

Second, the three types of victimization were then each separated into three variables, resulting in a total of nine dependent variables. Six of the nine variables were measured as dichotomous variables, and the other three were measured continuously. Verbal abuse was measured in the following manner: verbal abuse experienced in one's career (VERBAL—dichotomous dependent variable), verbal abuse experienced in the past 12 months (RECENT VERBAL—dichotomous dependent variable), and the frequency of verbal abuse experienced in the past 12 months (TOTAL VERBAL—continuous dependent variable). It should be noted that the third dependent variable was utilized for only those respondents who had reported verbal victimization. Threats of physical harm and physical acts of violence were measured in the same manner as verbal abuse (THREATS, RECENT THREATS, TOTAL THREATS, PHYSICAL, RECENT PHYSICAL, TOTAL PHYSICAL). The descriptive statistics for the nine dependent variables are presented in Table 4.

Table 4—Descriptive Statistics—Dependent Variables

| Variable | Mean | SD | N |
|---|---|---|---|
| VERBAL | 0.85 | 0.36 | 449 |
| THREATS | 0.55 | 0.50 | 449 |
| PHYSICAL | 0.52 | 0.50 | 449 |
| RECENT VERBAL | 0.75 | 0.43 | 449 |
| RECENT THREATS | 0.40 | 0.49 | 449 |
| RECENT PHYSCIAL | 0.35 | 0.48 | 449 |
| TOTAL VERBAL | 1.96 | 1.62 | 337 |
| TOTAL THREATS | 1.30 | 1.15 | 180 |
| TOTAL PHYSICAL | 1.57 | 1.65 | 157 |

The first three dichotomous dependent variables—verbal abuse (VERBAL), threats of physical harm (THREATS), and physical acts of violence (PHYSICAL) experienced in one's career—were coded as follows. If the employee never experienced any type of victimization, the variable was coded as a zero. If the employee did experience victimization, the variable was coded as a one. The mean score for VERBAL was .85, indicating that 85% of those surveyed experienced verbal abuse in their career. The mean score for THREATS was .55, which means that 55% of the respondents experienced threats of physical harm during their career. The mean score for PHYSICAL was .52, indicating that 52% of those surveyed had experienced physical acts of violence during their career.

The next set of dichotomous dependent variables— verbal abuse (RECENT VERBAL), threats of physical harm (RECENT THREATS), and physical acts of violence (RECENT PHYSICAL) experienced in the past 12 months—were coded the same way as the previous dependent variables (i.e., zero and one). The mean score for RECENT VERBAL was .75, indicating that 75% of those surveyed had experienced verbal abuse within the past year. The mean score for RECENT THREATS was .40, indicating that 40% of the respondents had experienced threats of physical harm within the past 12 months. The mean score for RECENT PHYSICAL was .35, which means that only 35% of those surveyed had experienced physical acts of violence within the past year.

The last set of dependent variables—the frequency of verbal abuse (TOTAL VERBAL), threats of physical harm (TOTAL THREATS), and physical acts of violence (TOTAL PHYSICAL) experienced in the past 12 months by those who had reported each type of victimization—were all coded continuously. Due to these dependent variables being positively skewed, the natural log of each was utilized. The range for TOTAL VERBAL was zero to 6.55, with a mean of 1.96. The range for TOTAL THREATS was zero to 5.30, with a mean of 1.30. Finally, the range for TOTAL PHYSICAL was zero to 6.22, with a mean of 1.57.

Overall, based on the information discussed above, the risk of violent victimization varied according to victimization type. While approximately 52% of those surveyed indicated that they had experienced a physical act of violence within their career, only 35% reported that they had experienced physical violence within the past 12 months. As for threats of violence, 55% of those surveyed reported experiencing these threats during their career. Within the past 12 months, approximately 40% reported experiencing threats. The pattern was the same for verbal abuse, but with greater levels of victimization reported. While 85% reported experiencing verbal abuse during their career, 75% reported experiencing verbal abuse in the past year. Finally among those respondents who reported being victimized in the past year, the frequency of verbal abuse was greater than the frequency of threats of physical harm and actual physical victimization.

## OLS & Logistic Regression Assumptions

The following addresses the ordinary least squares (OLS) and logistic regression assumptions. The OLS regression assumptions are considered first, followed by a discussion of logistic regression diagnostics. According to Lewis-Beck (1980), the bivariate OLS regression assumptions are as follows:

1.   No specification error.
     a.   The relationship between $X_i$ and $Y_i$ is linear.
     b.   No relevant independent variables have been excluded.
     c.   No irrelevant independent variables have been included.

2.   No measurement error.
     a.   The variables $X_i$ and $Y_i$ are accurately measured.

3.   The following assumptions concern the error term, $\in_i$:
     a.   Zero mean: $E(\in_i)=0$.
          i.   For each observation, the expected value of the error term is zero. (We use the symbol $E(\ )$ for the expected value which, for a random variable, is simply equal to its mean.)
     b.   Homoscedasticity: $E(\in_i^2)=6^2$.
          i.   The variance of the error term is constant for all values of $X_i$.
     c.   No autocorrelation: $E(\in_i \in_j)=0$ (i  j).
          i.   The error terms are uncorrelated.
     d.   The independent variable is uncorrelated with the error term:
          $E(\in_i X_i)=0$.
     e.   Normality.
          i.   The error term, $\in_i$, is normally distributed. (p. 26)

The first assumption to be addressed is specification error. The OLS models were checked to ensure that there was a linear relationship between the independent and dependent variables. First, individual scatterplots for the independent and dependent variables were visually inspected. If the assumption of linearity was met, it would be expected that these scatterplots would suggest a relatively straight line (Mertler & Vannatta, 2001). The individual scatterplots did not suggest a problem with nonlinearity. In addition, residual plots were also examined for all of the models, and these residual plots did not reveal a pattern indicative of nonlinearity.

Second, to make sure that no relevant independent variables were excluded, and that no irrelevant independent variables were included, a thorough review of the literature was conducted. Furthermore, a variety of multivariate models were employed in an effort to reduce specification error and identify significant variables. Qualitative interviews were also conducted, which provided feedback regarding the appropriateness of the variables.

The next assumption to be discussed concerns the issue of measurement error. This assumption provides that all independent and dependent variables are accurately measured. In addition to a thorough literature review that identified how variables related to routine activities theory have been measured in past research, qualitative interviews were also conducted to provide additional checks on the clarity of questionnaire items. Both the extensive literature review and initial qualitative interviews aided in minimizing measurement error.

The last set of assumptions pertains to the error term. First, the error term should have a mean of zero. According to Lewis-Beck (1980), "a zero mean is of little concern because, regardless, the least squares estimate of the slope is unchanged" (p. 28). However, checks of the residual statistics indicated that the means were all virtually zero, which satisfies this assumption.

Second, there should be homoscedasticity or a constant variance across the error term. To check for homoscedasticity, a visual inspection of the residual scatterplots was completed. In the linear models, the residuals were plotted fairly evenly around the reference line, which indicates that this assumption was met. If the points were not evenly scattered around the reference line, instead appearing in a fan-shaped pattern, this would have indicated the problem of heteroscedasticity (Mertler & Vannatta, 2001).

Third, there should be no autocorrelation, meaning that the residuals should not be correlated among themselves. According to Lewis-Beck (1980), "autocorrelation more frequently appears with time-series variables (repeated observations on the same unit through time) than cross-section variables (unique observations on different units at the same point in time)" (p. 28). Although this study did not involve time-series data, the Durbin-Watson statistic was used to check for the possibility of autocorrelation (Schroeder, Sjoquist, & Stephen, 1986). According to Pindyck and Rubinfeld (1981), a Durbin-Watson statistic near two indicates that there is not a problem with autocorrelation. In this case, all Durbin-Watson statistics were very near or slightly less than two (with a range from 1.530 to 1.933), indicating that autocorrelation was not present.

Fourth, the error term should not be correlated with any of the independent variables. According to Lewis-Beck (1980), "the simplest way to test for this violation is to evaluate the error term as a collection of excluded explanatory variables, each of which might be correlated with X" (p. 29). Therefore, if all relevant independent variables are incorporated into the model, this assumption will not be violated. If relevant independent variables are excluded, the assumption must be trusted that the excluded variables are not highly correlated with the independent variables actually in the model. Again, every effort was made in this study (through the literature review and the qualitative research) to ensure a properly specified model with accurately measured variables.

The last assumption regarding the error term is normality. In other words, the error term should be normally distributed. According to Lewis-Beck (1980), a normally distributed error term would be indicated by a frequency distribution that exemplifies a normal or bell-shaped curve, with less than 5% of the cases in the tails. To check for normality, casewise diagnostics were utilized to see if the residuals were normally distributed. In all cases, the casewise diagnostics showed that less than 4% of the cases or outliers fell in the tails. Also, a visual inspection of residual histograms showed a bell-shape curve. It should also be noted that the natural log of the continuous dependent variables was employed, since the distribution of a continuous dependent variable and the corresponding error term is essentially the same (only their means are different), and using the natural log corrected for a positive skew.

There is also one other assumption that must be noted in addition to the bivariate regression assumptions listed above. Since this study involved multivariate analyses, there must be no problem with multicollinearity (Menard, 1995). Multicollinearity occurs when two or more independent variables are highly correlated with one another. In other words, they have something in common (Bachman & Paternoster, 1997). In order to check for multicollinearity, the following statistics were examined: bivariate correlations among the independent variables, tolerance statistics, and variance inflation factors.

An inspection of the bivariate correlation matrix showed that there were only three zero-order correlations greater than $\pm.50$ [AGE and EXPERIENCE (.558); NONRESIDENTIAL and RESIDENTIAL facilities (-.554); URBAN and SUBURBAN (-.612)]. According to Bachman and Paternoster (1997), multicollinearity should not pose a problem if the coefficients are below $\pm.70$. In this case, none of the correlations were higher than $\pm.70$, thus it did not appear that there were any problems with multicollinearity.

However, to ensure that multicollinearity was not a problem, further checks were done by examining tolerance statistics and variance inflation factors from linear probability models. Tolerance is another way to assess multicollinearity that may exist among independent variables. Tolerance statistics range from zero to one. Tolerances closer to zero indicate multicollinearity, whereas tolerances closer to one indicate that the variables are independent from one another (Mertler & Vannatta, 2001). An inspection of these statistics showed that all tolerances were greater than .50. Recommendations vary, but according to Menard (1995), tolerances of less than .20 indicate a problem. Mertler and Vannatta (2001) suggest that tolerances of less than .10 indicate a problem. In this case, there did not appear to be a problem with multicollinearity, as the tolerances were all greater than .50 and exceed the recommended guidelines.

Variance inflation factors are another technique for assessing multicollinearity. Mertler and Vannatta (2001, p. 169) cite Steven (1992) as stating that, "the variance inflation factor for a given predictor indicates whether there exists a strong linear association between it and all remaining predictors." In this study, all variance inflation factors were less than 2.0. It has been suggested that variance inflation factors equaling 10 or higher are an indicator of a multicollinearity problem (Mertler & Vannatta, 2001). In this case, the variance inflation factors of less than 2.0 are well below the recommended guidelines. Thus, based on these checks, multicollinearity was not a problem.

Logistic regression was also utilized in this study because using OLS regression with dichotomous dependent variables would violate a number of the assumptions discussed above. Since logistic regression uses maximum likelihood estimation, problems associated with using OLS with dichotomous dependent variables are eliminated (Menard, 1995). Such problems include heteroscedasticity, nonlinearity, a nonnormal error term, and predicted probabilities beyond 1.0.

Upon examination of the first two regression assumptions, pertaining to specification error and measurement error, neither appeared to be a problem. Linearity was not an issue, since logistic regression is designed to deal with nonlinear relationships involving dichotomous dependent variables. In order to reduce the possibility of specification error, a number of multivariate models were employed to identify significant variables. Conducting a thorough literature review, which ensured that all relevant independent variables were included, and that no irrelevant independent variables were included, minimized both specification error and measurement error. In addition, the qualitative interviews provided further verification that these assumptions were satisfied.

As for the assumptions concerning the error term, logistic regression corrects for the violations that would normally take place when using a dichotomous dependent variable in OLS regression. However, there is still a concern regarding the number of cases that reside in the tails of the residual distribution. These outliers or influential cases must be investigated to make sure that they are not producing a major impact on the findings of the model. In this study, there was a low percentage of residuals in the tails of the distributions (i.e., less than 5% in all models). However, to provide a further check on the models, the extreme outliers were eliminated and the models were rerun. No significant changes in the findings were noted overall. Thus, the original models were reported and discussed.

Last, since the logistic regression models involved multivariate analyses, multicollinearity is also a possible concern. As was stated previously, bivariate correlations, tolerance statistics, and variance inflation factors were all examined.

## Multivariate Results

This section presents the multivariate findings, based on the nine dependent variables. The results are presented according to type of victimization: verbal abuse, threats of violence, and physical acts of violence. Four major models were initially constructed for each one of the dependent variables in order to examine the victimization and to check for consistency across the models. Since all of the models produced similar findings, only the findings of the original model are reported and discussed.

## Verbal Abuse

The first type of victimization examined was verbal abuse. As stated previously, this dependent variable was measured in the following three ways: verbal abuse experienced in one's career (VERBAL—dichotomous dependent variable), verbal abuse experienced in the past 12 months (RECENT VERBAL—dichotomous dependent variable), and all incidents of verbal abuse experienced in the past 12 months (TOTAL VERBAL—continuous dependent variable).

Upon examination of verbal abuse experienced in one's career (VERBAL), the results of the full logistic model indicated that the following independent variables were significant at the .05 level: SCHIZOPHRENIA, TRAINING, EDUCATION, and HOURS. The Cox and Snell R-square was .162, and the Nagelkerke R-square was .287, suggesting that this model explained 16.2% to 28.7% of the variation in the dependent variable VERBAL. All of the coefficients were positive. See Table 5.

The coefficient for the variable SCHIZOPHRENIA, which provides a measure of exposure to potential offenders, indicates that experiences of verbal abuse were found to be more likely among those employees regularly working with schizophrenic clients (b=.754; p=<.05). The variables TRAINING and EDUCATION provide measures of target suitability. Both had positive coefficients, which suggests that experiences of verbal abuse were more likely among those mental health workers with more training (b=.076; p=<.05) and education (b=.293; p=<.05). As will be later discussed, some of the qualitative interviews suggested that the more training and education an employee receives on crisis intervention and violence prevention, the greater the awareness level. It may be that those with more training and education are more likely to recognize victimization and thus are more likely to report the victimization. Finally, the last variable, HOURS, was also a measure of target suitability. The coefficient again was positive (b=.057; p=<.01), which indicates that employees working more hours during the week experienced more verbal abuse.

Table 5: Logistic Regression Estimates For Verbal Abuse Experienced In One's Career—Full Model (N=391)

| Variable | B (SE) | Wald | Exp(B) |
|---|---|---|---|
| DANGER | .092(.066) | 1.943 | 1.096 |
| CLIENT # | .022 (.012) | 3.451 | 1.023 |
| SCHIZOPHRENIA | .754 (.379) | 3.963* | 2.125 |
| SUBSTANCE ABUSE | .125 (.356) | .124 | 1.134 |
| SUBURBAN | .355 (.409) | .756 | 1.426 |
| URBAN | .528 (.418) | 1.596 | 1.695 |
| # COWORKERS | -.009 (.013) | .550 | .991 |
| NONRESIDENTIAL | -.502 (.416) | 1.455 | .605 |
| RESIDENTIAL | .210(.502) | .175 | 1.234 |
| TRAINING | .076(.035) | 4.737* | 1.079 |
| EDUCATION | .293(.131) | 4.982* | 1.340 |
| EXPERIENCE | .060(.031) | 3.771 | 1.062 |
| AGE | .000(.016) | .000 | 1.000 |
| GENDER | -.502(.406) | 1.533 | .605 |
| STYLE | -.028(.036) | .618 | .972 |
| DRUGS | .499(.414) | 1.453 | 1.647 |
| HOURS | .057(.020) | 7.607** | 1.058 |
| DAY | -.686(.386) | 3.160 | .504 |
| Constant | -2.750 (1.230) | 4.997 | .064 |
| Log Likelihood: 255.694** | | | |
| Cox & Snell $R^2$ : .162 | | | |
| Nagelkerke $R^2$ : .287 | | | |

*p<.05  **p<.01

The results of the full logistic model for verbal abuse experienced in the past 12 months (RECENT VERBAL) indicated that the following independent variables were significant at the .05 level: CLIENT#, SCHIZOPHRENIA, URBAN, TRAINING, GENDER, HOURS, and DAY. The Cox and Snell R-square was .192, and the Nagelkerke R-square was .283, suggesting that this model explained 19.2% to 28.3% of the variation in the dependent variable RECENT VERBAL. See Table 6.

Table 6: Logistic Regression Estimates For Recent Verbal Abuse Experienced In Past 12 Months—Full Model (N=391)

| Variable | B (SE) | Wald | Exp(B) |
|---|---|---|---|
| DANGER | .005 (.028) | .029 | 1.005 |
| CLIENT # | .026 (.008) | 9.396** | 1.026 |
| SCHIZOPHRENIA | .632 (.307) | 4.223* | 1.880 |
| SUBSTANCE ABUSE | .243 (.294) | .683 | 1.275 |
| SUBURBAN | .257 (.328) | .613 | 1.293 |
| URBAN | .767 (.352) | 4.749* | 2.153 |
| # COWORKERS | .000 (.011) | .002 | 1.000 |
| NONRESIDENTIAL | -.627 (.345) | 3.306 | .534 |
| RESIDENTIAL | -.267 (.394) | .458 | .766 |
| TRAINING | .046 (.022) | 4.472* | 1.047 |
| EDUCATION | .101 (.107) | .901 | 1.106 |
| EXPERIENCE | -.013 (.022) | .345 | .987 |
| AGE | .003 (.014) | .037 | 1.003 |
| GENDER | -.977 (.339) | 8.327** | .376 |
| STYLE | .115 (.064) | 3.252 | 1.122 |
| DRUGS | .157 (.320) | .241 | 1.170 |
| HOURS | .054 (.018) | 9.018** | 1.056 |
| DAY | -.815 (.314) | 6.729** | .443 |
| Constant | -1.961 (1.104) | 3.156 | .141 |
| Log Likelihood: 359.347** | | | |
| Cox & Snell R$^2$: .192 | | | |
| Nagelkerke R$^2$:  .283 | | | |

*p<.05   **p<.01

Coefficients for CLIENT# (b=.026; p=<.01), SCHIZOPHRENIA (b=.632; p=<.05), and URBAN (b=.767; p=<.05), all measures of exposure to potential offenders, were positive. This indicates that those mental health workers who had more client contacts on a weekly basis, worked regularly with schizophrenics, and worked in an urban environment were more likely to experience verbal abuse in the past 12 months.

The last four variables, TRAINING, GENDER, HOURS, and DAY were measures of target suitability. TRAINING had a positive coefficient (b=.046; p=<.05). This again indicates that employees with more training were more likely to experience verbal abuse in the past year. GENDER (b= -.977; p=<.01) and DAY (b= -.815; p=<.01) had negative coefficients, indicating that males and those regularly working the evening or night shift were more likely to experience verbal abuse in the past 12 months. The variable HOURS had a positive coefficient (b=.054; p=<.01), which again suggests that those who worked more hours during the week were more likely to experience verbal abuse during the past year.

The results of the full linear model examining total verbal abuse experienced in the past 12 months (TOTAL VERBAL) indicated that the following independent variables were significant at the .05 level: DANGER, SUBSTANCE ABUSE, TRAINING, and DRUGS. See Table 7. It should be noted that this model was based only on those respondents who reported being verbally victimized during the past 12 months. The adjusted R-square was .102, suggesting that this linear model only explained 10.2% of the variation in the dependent variable TOTAL VERBAL.

The first two variables, DANGER and SUBSTANCE ABUSE, were measures of exposure to potential offenders. DANGER (b=.056; p<.01) had a positive coefficient, indicating that, among those who were victimized, employees who perceived more of their weekly client contacts to be dangerous experienced a higher frequency of verbal abuse. SUBSTANCE ABUSE (b= -.440;p<.05) had a negative coefficient, which suggests that, among those who were victimized, employees who worked regularly with substance abusers experienced a lower frequency of verbal abuse.

TRAINING, a measure of target suitability, had a positive coefficient (b=.022; p=<.05), suggesting that, among employees who were victimized, those who had more training experienced a greater frequency of verbal abuse. The last significant variable, DRUGS, was also a measure of target suitability. DRUGS had a positive coefficient (b=.513; p<.05), which indicates that, among those who were victimized, employees having access to or carrying drugs experienced a greater frequency of verbal abuse.

Table 7: OLS Regression Estimates For The Natural Log Of Total Recent Verbal Abuse Experienced In Past 12 Months—Full Model (N=292)

| Variable | B (SE) | T Score | Beta |
|---|---|---|---|
| DANGER | .056 (.017) | 3.295** | .200 |
| CLIENT # | .004 (.003) | 1.246 | .078 |
| SCHIZOPHRENIA | -.341 (.227) | -1.502 | -.100 |
| SUBSTANCE ABUSE | -.440 (.198) | -2.219* | -.131 |
| SUBURBAN | .137 (.255) | .536 | .041 |
| URBAN | .184 (.255) | .722 | .056 |
| # COWORKERS | -.002 (.007) | -3.49 | -.020 |
| NONRESIDENTIAL | -.262 (.253) | -1.035 | -.074 |
| RESIDENTIAL | .049 (.252) | .198 | .015 |
| TRAINING | .021 (010) | 2.136* | .126 |
| EDUCATION | -.021 (.076) | -.284 | -.020 |
| EXPERIENCE | -.008 (.015) | -.560 | -.040 |
| AGE | .009 (.009) | .969 | .067 |
| GENDER | .065 (.201) | -.328 | -.019 |
| STYLE | .010 (.021) | .506 | .029 |
| DRUGS | .513 (.217) | 2.361* | .154 |
| HOURS | .007 (.012) | .623 | .036 |
| DAY | -.142 (.198) | -.718 | -.043 |
| Constant: | 1.265 (.806) | 1.569 | |
| Adjusted R Square: .102 | | | |
| F Score: 2.829** | | | |

*p<.05   **p<.01

# Threats

The second dependent variable, threats of violence, was also measured in the same three ways as verbal abuse [i.e., threats experienced in one's career (THREATS—dichotomous dependent variable), threats experienced in the past 12 months (RECENT THREATS—dichotomous dependent variable), and total incidents of threats experienced in the past 12 months (TOTAL THREATS—continuous dependent variable).

The results of the full logistic model for all threats experienced in one's career indicated that the following independent variables were significant at the .05 level: DANGER, NONRESIDENTIAL, EXPERIENCE, AGE, GENDER, HOURS, and DAY. The Cox and Snell R-square was .228, and the Nagelkerke R-square was .306, suggesting that this model explained 22.8% to 30.6% of the variation in the dependent variable THREATS. See Table 8.

The variable DANGER provided a measure of exposure to potential offenders. DANGER (b=.091; p<.05) had a positive coefficient, which indicates that experiences of threats were found to be more likely among those employees who perceived more of their weekly client contacts to be dangerous.

The variable, NONRESIDENTIAL, provided a measure of guardianship. NONRESIDENTIAL (b= -.608; p=.05) had a negative coefficient, suggesting that those who work in nonresidential facilities were less likely to experience threats than those working in crisis and residential facilities.

EXPERIENCE (b=.103; p<.01), AGE (b= -.025; p<.05), GENDER (b= -.729; p<.01), HOURS (b=.047; p<.01), and DAY (b= -.731; p<.01) all provided measures of target suitability. EXPERIENCE and HOURS had positive coefficients, which suggests that employees with more experience in the field were more likely to experience threats and employees working more hours were more likely to experience threats. AGE, GENDER, and DAY had negative coefficients, which indicates that younger employees, males, and those working evening or night shifts were more likely to experience threats.

Table 8: Logistic Regression Estimates For Threats Experienced In One's Career—Full Model (N=391)

| Variable | B (SE) | Wald | Exp (B) |
|---|---|---|---|
| DANGER | .091 (.037) | 6.188* | 1.096 |
| CLIENT # | .001 (.005) | .056 | 1.001 |
| SCHIZOPHRENIA | .440 (.276) | 2.536 | 1.552 |
| SUBSTANCE ABUSE | -.414 (.257) | 2.604 | .661 |
| SUBURBAN | .608 (.312) | 1.394 | 1.838 |
| URBAN | .375 (.318) | 1.394 | 1.455 |
| # COWORKERS | -.007 (.009) | .611 | .993 |
| NONRESIDENTIAL | -.608 (.310) | 3.851* | .544 |
| RESIDENTIAL | -.452 (.341) | 1.757 | .637 |
| TRAINING | .030 (.016) | 3.494 | 1.030 |
| EDUCATION | -.03 (.096) | .001 | .997 |
| EXPERIENCE | .103 (.022) | 22.120** | 1.109 |
| AGE | -.025 (.012) | 3.978* | .976 |
| GENDER | -.729 (.271) | 7.218** | .482 |
| STYLE | .105 (.058) | 3.263 | 1.110 |
| DRUGS | .351 (.285) | 1.516 | 1.420 |
| HOURS | .047 (.017) | 8.001** | 1.048 |
| DAY | -.731 (.264) | 7.644** | .482 |
| Constant: | -1.599 (1.019) | 2.465 | .202 |
| Log Likelihood: 433.759** | | | |
| Cox & Snell $R^2$ : .228 | | | |
| Nagelkerke $R^2$ : .306 | | | |

*p<.05   **p<.01

The results of the full logistic model examining threats experienced in the past 12 months (RECENT THREATS) indicated that the following independent variables were significant at the .05 level: DANGER, NONRESIDENTIAL, RESIDENTIAL, GENDER, STYLE, HOURS, and DAY. The Cox and Snell R-square was .205, and the Nagelkerke R-square was .277, suggesting that this model explained 20.5% to 27.7% of the variation in the dependent variable RECENT THREATS. See Table 9.

Table 9: Logistic Regression Estimates For Recent Threats Experienced In Past 12 Months—Full Model (N=391)

| Variable | B (SE) | Wald | Exp (B) |
|---|---|---|---|
| DANGER | .051 (.024) | 4.526* | 1.053 |
| CLIENT # | .008 (.005) | 2.535 | 1.008 |
| SCHIZOPHRENIA | -.023(.278) | .007 | .978 |
| SUBSTANCE ABUSE | .023 (.253) | .008 | 1.023 |
| SUBURBAN | .115 (.313) | .136 | 1.122 |
| URBAN | .193 (.321) | .360 | 1.212 |
| # COWORKERS | -.009 (.009) | 1.082 | .991 |
| NONRESIDENTIAL | -.749 (.309) | 5.859* | .473 |
| RESIDENTIAL | -.965 (.339) | 8.108** | .381 |
| TRAINING | .012 (.014) | .774 | 1.012 |
| EDUCATION | -.116 (.094) | 1.517 | .890 |
| EXPERIENCE | .029 (.020) | 2.084 | 1.029 |
| AGE | -.020 (.013) | 2.478 | .980 |
| GENDER | -1.062(.263) | 16.256** | .346 |
| STYLE | .187 (.056) | 11.009** | 1.205 |
| DRUGS | .368 (.278) | 1.759 | 1.445 |
| HOURS | .037 (.017) | 5.123* | 1.038 |
| DAY | -.879 (.256) | 11.817** | .415 |
| Constant: | -.468 (1.011) | .214 | .626 |
| Log Likelihood: 439.239** | | | |
| Cox & Snell $R^2$ : .205 | | | |
| Nagelkerke $R^2$ : .277 | | | |

*p<.05   **p<.01

DANGER (b=.051; p<.05) provided a measure of exposure to potential offenders and had a positive coefficient. This indicates that employees who viewed more of their weekly client contacts as dangerous were more likely to experience threats.

NONRESIDENTIAL (b= -.749; p<.05) and RESIDENTIAL (b= -.965; p<.01) provided measures of guardianship. Both had negative coefficients, which suggests that those who work in crisis facilities were more likely to experience threats than those working in nonresidential or residential facilities.

The rest of the variables, GENDER, STYLE, HOURS, and DAY, all provided measures of target suitability. GENDER (b= -1.062; p<.01) had a negative coefficient, which suggests that males were more likely to experience threats than females. STYLE (b=.187; p<.01) had a positive coefficient, which indicates that those who reported having a more firm and assertive style were more likely to experience threats. HOURS (b=.037; p<.05) had a positive coefficient, which suggests that employees who work more hours were more likely to experience threats. The last variable, DAY (b= -.879; p<.01), had a negative coefficient, which indicates that those who regularly work evening or night shifts were more likely to experience threats.

The results of the full linear model examining total threats experienced in the past 12 months (TOTAL THREATS) indicated that the following independent variables were significant at the .05 level: DANGER, SCHIZOPHRENIA, and SUBSTANCE ABUSE. This model was based on only those respondents who reported being threatened during the past 12 months. The adjusted R-square was .12, suggesting that this linear model only explained 12% of the variation in the dependent variable TOTAL THREATS. See Table 10.

All three of the significant variables provide measures for exposure to potential offenders. The coefficient for DANGER (b=.036; p<.05) was positive. This indicates that, among those who were victimized, employees who perceived more of their weekly client contacts to be dangerous experienced a greater frequency of threats. Both of the coefficients for SCHIZOPHRENIA (b= -.516; p<.05) and SUBSTANCE ABUSE (b= -.722; p<.01) were negative, suggesting that, among those who were victimized, employees who reported working regularly with clients suffering from these disorders experienced a lower frequency of threats.

Table 10: OLS Regression Estimates For The Natural Log Of Total Recent Threats Experienced In Past 12 Months—Full Model (N=160)

| Variable | B (SE) | T Score | Beta |
|---|---|---|---|
| DANGER | .035 (.014) | 2.557 | .205 |
| CLIENT # | .001 (.003) | .516 | .046 |
| SCHIZOPHRENIA | -.516 (.211) | -2.450* | -.212 |
| SUBSTANCE ABUSE | -.722 (.192) | -3.758** | -.303 |
| SUBURBAN | .026 (.248) | .106 | .011 |
| URBAN | .206 (.252) | .817 | .087 |
| # COWORKERS | .005 (.007) | .759 | .060 |
| NONRESIDENTIAL | -.337 (.424) | -1.392 | -.129 |
| RESIDENTIAL | .075 (.248) | .304 | .031 |
| TRAINING | .012 (.009) | 1.303 | .107 |
| EDUCATION | .000 (.072) | -.010 | -.001 |
| EXPERIENCE | -.007 (.016) | -.484 | -.048 |
| AGE | -.006 (.010) | -.585 | -.056 |
| GENDER | -.189 (.186) | -1.014 | -.079 |
| STYLE | .018 (.016) | 1.138 | .090 |
| DRUGS | .219 (.208) | 1.049 | .093 |
| HOURS | .011 (.013) | .873 | .072 |
| DAY | -.052 (.195) | -.217 | -.023 |
| Constant: | 1.343 (.806) | 1.666 | |
| Adjusted R Square: .120 | | | |
| F Score: 2.208** | | | |

*p<.05  **p<.01

## Physical Acts

The third dependent variable, physical acts of violence, was also measured the same way as verbal abuse and threats [i.e., physical acts of violence experienced in one's career (PHYSICAL—dichotomous dependent variable), physical acts of violence experienced in the past 12 months (RECENT PHYSICAL—dichotomous dependent variable), and all incidents of physical acts of violence experienced in the past 12 months (TOTAL PHYSICAL—continuous dependent variable)].

The results of the full logistic model examining physical acts experienced in one's career (PHYSICAL) indicated that the following independent variables were significant at the .05 level: DANGER, RESIDENTIAL, EXPERIENCE, and HOURS. The Cox and Snell R-square was .183, and the Nagelkerke R-square was .245, suggesting that this model explained 18.3% to 24.5% of the variation in the dependent variable PHYSICAL. See Table 11.

Table 11:  Logistic Regression Estimates For Physical Victimization Experienced In One's Career—Full Model (N=391)

| Variable | B (SE) | Wald | Exp (B) |
|---|---|---|---|
| DANGER | .152 (.042) | 12.894** | 1.164 |
| CLIENT # | .002 (.005) | .210 | 1.002 |
| SCHIZOPHRENIA | -.103(.267) | .149 | .902 |
| SUBSTANCE ABUSE | -.132 (.246) | .287 | .877 |
| SUBURBAN | .419 (.300) | 1.950 | 1.521 |
| URBAN | .376 (.307) | 1.505 | 1.457 |
| # COWORKERS | -.010 (.009) | 1.248 | .990 |
| NONRESIDENTIAL | -.445 (.299) | 2.209 | .641 |
| RESIDENTIAL | -.709 (.326) | 4.721* | .492 |
| TRAINING | .007 (.014) | .232 | 1.007 |
| EDUCATION | -.086 (.092) | .862 | .918 |
| EXPERIENCE | .065 (.020) | 10.852** | 1.068 |
| AGE | -.009 (.012) | .524 | .991 |
| GENDER | -.150 (.25) | .347 | .861 |
| STYLE | .060 (.052) | 1.326 | 1.062 |
| DRUGS | -.089 (.273) | .107 | .914 |
| HOURS | .055 (.016) | 11.337** | 1.056 |
| DAY | -.445 (.252) | 3.126 | .641 |
| Constant: | -1.934 (.993) | 3.794 | .145 |
| Log Likelihood: 461.581** | | | |
| Cox & Snell $R^2$ : .183 | | | |
| Nagelkerke $R^2$ : .245 | | | |

*p<.05   **p<.01

DANGER provided a measure for exposure to potential offenders. DANGER (b=.152; p<.01) had a positive coefficient, indicating that employees who perceived more of their weekly client contacts to be dangerous were more likely to experience physical acts of violence. RESIDENTIAL provided a measure of guardianship. RESIDENTIAL (b= -.709; p=<.05) had a negative coefficient, which suggests that workers in residential facilities were less likely to experience physical acts of violence than employees who worked in a residential or crisis setting.

The variables EXPERIENCE and HOURS provided measures of target suitability. EXPERIENCE (b=.065; p<.01) had a positive coefficient, which indicates that employees with more experience were more likely to encounter physical acts of violence. The coefficient for HOURS (b=.055; p<.01) was positive, which indicates that employees who worked more hours were more likely to experience physical acts of violence. Another variable worth noting is DAY, which had a p-value of .077. This provides suggestive evidence that there may be a relationship between this independent variable and the dependent variable. The negative coefficient suggests that employees who regularly worked during the day were less likely to experience physical victimization.

The results of the full logistic model examining physical acts experienced in the past 12 months (RECENT PHYSICAL) indicated that the following independent variables were significant at the .05 level: DANGER, TRAINING, DAY, and HOURS. The Cox and Snell R-square was .104, and the Nagelkerke R-square was .143, suggesting that this model only explained 10.4% to 14.3% of the variation in the dependent variable RECENT PHYSICAL. See Table 12.

The variable DANGER provided a measure for exposure to potential offenders. The coefficient for DANGER (b=.051; p<.05) was positive, which suggests that those employees who perceived more of their weekly client contacts to be dangerous were more likely to experience physical acts of violence.

The last three variables, TRAINING, DAY and HOURS, provided measures of target suitability. TRAINING (b=.032; p<.05) had a positive coefficient, indicating that the more training an employee had in the past year, the more likely they were to experience physical victimization. The coefficient for DAY (b= -.647; p<.01) was negative, which suggests that those who regularly worked during the evening or at night were at greater risk of encountering physical acts of violence. The coefficient for HOURS (b=.047; p<.01) was positive, which suggests that the more hours an employee worked, the greater the likelihood of physical victimization.

Table 12: Logistic Regression Estimates For Recent Physical Victimization Experienced In Past 12 Months—Full Model (N=391)

| Variable | B (SE) | Wald | Exp (B) |
|---|---|---|---|
| DANGER | .051 (.022) | 5.495* | 1.054 |
| CLIENT # | -.002 (.005) | .168 | .998 |
| SCHIZOPHRENIA | -.252 (.269) | .883 | .777 |
| SUBSTANCE ABUSE | -.313 (.250) | 1.574 | .731 |
| SUBURBAN | .010 (.303) | .001 | 1.010 |
| URBAN | -.051 (.309) | .027 | .950 |
| # COWORKERS | -.003 (.008) | .158 | 1.003 |
| NONRESIDENTIAL | -.325 (.303) | 1.156 | .722 |
| RESIDENTIAL | -.207 (.323) | .410 | .813 |
| TRAINING | .032 (.013) | 5.652* | 1.032 |
| EDUCATION | -.050 (.092) | .299 | .951 |
| EXPERIENCE | .007 (.019) | .152 | 1.008 |
| AGE | -.009 (.012) | .543 | .991 |
| GENDER | -.077 (.255) | .091 | .926 |
| STYLE | -.009 (.031) | .074 | .992 |
| DRUGS | -.039 (.270) | .021 | .962 |
| HOURS | .047 (.016) | 8.644** | 1.048 |
| DAY | -.647 (.246) | 6.898** | .524 |
| Constant: | -1.314 (.962) | 1.868 | .269 |
| Log Likelihood: 462.480** | | | |
| Cox & Snell $R^2$ : .104 | | | |
| Nagelkerke $R^2$ : .143 | | | |

*p<.05   **p<.01

The results of the full linear model examining total physical acts experienced in the past 12 months (TOTAL PHYSICAL) indicated that the following independent variables were significant at the .05 level: DANGER, SCHIZOPHRENIA, and STYLE. This model was based on only those respondents who reported being physically victimized during the past 12 months. The adjusted R-square was .192, suggesting that this linear model explained 19.2% of the variation in the dependent variable TOTAL PHYSICAL. See Table 13.

Table 13: OLS Regression Estimates For The Natural Log Of Total Recent Physical Victimization Experienced In Past 12 Months—Full Model (N=136)

| Variable | B (SE) | T Score | Beta |
|---|---|---|---|
| DANGER | .042 (.019) | 2.208* | .187 |
| CLIENT # | .003 (.006) | .710 | .064 |
| SCHIZOPHRENIA | -1.264 (.303) | -4.177** | -.386 |
| SUBSTANCE ABUSE | -.166 (.294) | -.563 | -.048 |
| SUBURBAN | -.251 (.379) | -.663 | -.076 |
| URBAN | -.243 (.371) | -.657 | -.074 |
| # COWORKERS | -.005 (.011) | -.486 | -.044 |
| NONRESIDENTIAL | -.135 (.351) | -.385 | -.039 |
| RESIDENTIAL | -.449 (.417) | -1.077 | -.133 |
| TRAINING | .009 (.013) | .747 | .061 |
| EDUCATION | -.032 (.109) | -.299 | -.030 |
| EXPERIENCE | -.022 (.023) | -.330 | -.104 |
| AGE | -.020 (.014) | -1.512 | -.146 |
| GENDER | -.266 (.299) | -.891 | -.075 |
| STYLE | .163 (.067) | 2.442* | .210 |
| DRUGS | .350 (.322) | 1.086 | .106 |
| HOURS | .007 (.019) | .410 | .037 |
| DAY | -.539 (.290) | -1.856 | -.166 |
| Constant: | 2.777 (1.242) | 2.236 | |
| Adjusted R Square: .192 | | | |
| F Score: 2.780** | | | |

*p<.05  **p<.01

The variables DANGER and SCHIZOPHRENIA provided measures for exposure to potential offenders. The coefficient for DANGER (b=.042; p<.05) was positive, which suggests that, among those who were victimized, employees who perceived more of their weekly client contacts to be dangerous experienced a greater frequency of physical victimization. The coefficient for SCHIZOPHRENIA (b= -1.26; p<.01) was negative, which suggests that, among those who were victimized, employees who worked regularly with schizophrenics experienced a lesser frequency of physical victimization.

The variable STYLE provided a measure for target suitability. The coefficient for STYLE (b=.163; p<.05) was positive, which suggests that, among those who were victimized, employees who were more assertive and firm with their clients experienced a greater frequency of physical violence. The variable DAY should also be noted, as the p-value was .066. This provides suggestive evidence that there may be a relationship between the variable DAY and the dependent variable. The negative coefficient suggests that, among those who were victimized, employees who worked during the day experienced a lesser frequency of physical violence.

## Hypotheses

Based on the findings from the logistic and linear regression models presented above, this section addresses the 12 hypotheses introduced in Chapter III. Using these hypotheses, potential relationships between the three elements of routine activities theory—exposure to potential offenders, guardianship, and target suitability—and victimization at work were examined. The null hypotheses were that no significant differences or effects existed. The first four alternative hypotheses addressed the concept of exposure to potential offenders. The next two hypotheses examined the concept of guardianship. The last six hypotheses looked at the concept of target suitability.

## Potential Offenders

Some studies have shown that certain types of mentally ill patients or clients are more prone to violence than others (Arango et al., 1999; Link et al., 1992; Modestin & Ammann, 1996; Taylor et al., 1998; Wessely et al., 1994). Higher rates of violence have also been associated with more acute mental illness (Modestin & Ammann, 1996). For example, clients having dual diagnoses or schizophrenia have been found to have a greater propensity towards violence than clients with other diagnoses. Based on this literature, the following hypotheses were explored:

Ha(1): Employees working with the more severe mentally ill are more likely and more often victimized by those clients than employees working with the less severe mentally ill.

Ha(2): Employees who perceive greater danger on the part of their clients are more likely and more often victimized.

While the literature has indicated that working with clients suffering from more acute mental illness may put one at greater risk, the findings from this study simply do not support this overall view. In fact, only the likelihood of verbal victimization was found to be consistently higher among those employees working regularly with schizophrenics. On the other hand, among those who were threatened or physically victimized, working regularly with schizophrenics had a negative impact on the frequency of this victimization. This would indicate that workers experienced a lesser frequency of threats and physical victimization when working with schizophrenics as compared to working with other types of clients.

In addition, the qualitative interviews supported these findings, as many of the interviewees suggested that specific diagnoses were not significantly associated with a greater propensity towards violence. Rather, other factors may play a greater role in contributing to violent victimization. As such, the weight of the evidence would suggest that working with clients with more severe mental illness does not significantly increase one's risk or frequency of victimization, except for the experience of verbal victimization among those employees regularly working with schizophrenics. As such, there does not appear to be strong support for alternative hypothesis #1.

As for perceptions of danger, the findings showed that employees who viewed more of their weekly client contacts as dangerous reported a higher risk and frequency of victimization. In fact, DANGER was found to be significant among seven of the nine full models. Based on these findings, it would seem that there is fairly strong support for alternative hypothesis #2. Therefore, the null hypothesis is rejected, as there is a significant difference in victimization between those who perceived more of their weekly client contacts to be dangerous and those who perceived fewer of their weekly client contacts as dangerous. The literature has indicated that the following exposure factors also play a role in workplace victimization. They include working with capricious individuals (i.e., in health care, social service, or criminal justice settings) and working in crime-prone areas (LaMar et al., 1998; Nigro & Waugh, 1996; NIOSH, 1993a, NIOSH, 1993b; NIOSH, 1996; Warshaw & Messite, 1996). As such, the following hypotheses were explored:

Ha(3):    The greater the number of clients interacted with on a regular basis, the greater the likelihood and frequency of victimization by clients.

Ha(4):    Employees working in urban settings are more likely and more often victimized by clients than those working in rural and suburban settings.

While the literature has indicated that working with capricious individuals may put one at greater risk, the findings from this study do not support this viewpoint. In fact, only verbal victimization was found to be significantly higher among those employees having more weekly client contacts. Thus, there does not appear to be strong support for alternative hypothesis #3.

As for the environment in which one is employed, the literature has indicated that the type of community in which one works is related to risk of victimization (LaMar et al., 1998; Nigro & Waugh, 1996; NIOSH, 1993a; NIOSH, 1993b; NIOSH, 1996; Warshaw & Messite, 1996). For example, it is expected that crime rates would be higher in urban areas as opposed to rural and suburban areas. Thus, it would be expected that persons working in a nonurban environment would experience less victimization. Based on the quantitative findings, only verbal victimization was found to be higher among those employees who worked in an urban environment. As such, the weight of the evidence would suggest that working in an urban environment does not significantly increase one's risk or frequency of victimization, except for the experience of verbal victimization. Therefore, it does not appear that there is strong support for alternative hypothesis #4.

# Guardianship

Upon examination of the concept of guardianship, it is important to consider the environment in which one is employed. According to Warshaw and Messite (1996), "the risk varies with the environment: hospitalized patients, even though they tend to be more severely ill, are perhaps less likely to be violent because of the supervision, care, medication, and support they receive, as compared with those who have been deinstitutionalized and must cope with the stresses of living at home and in the community" (p. 996). Thus, depending on the workplace setting, employees may also be more at risk. As such, the following hypothesis was explored:

> Ha(5): Employees working in crisis programs are more likely and more often victimized by clients than those working in nonresidential or residential programs.

Based on the quantitative findings, the type of facility in which the employee worked had a significant impact on victimization, particularly with regard to threats and physical victimization. For example, those employees working in nonresidential or residential facilities were less likely overall to experience threats than those who worked in crisis facilities. In addition, those working in residential facilities were less likely to experience physical victimization in their career as compared to those working in crisis facilities. Based on these findings, there is support for alternative hypothesis #5. It appears that employees working in crisis facilities have a greater likelihood of being threatened by clients than those working in nonresidential and residential facilities, and working in crisis facilities tended to have a fairly consistent positive impact on victimization in the other models as well. As such, the null hypothesis is rejected, as there were differences in victimization depending on the type of facility in which one worked.

The literature also has indicated that working solely or in small groups may also play a role in workplace victimization (LaMar et al., 1998; Nigro & Waugh, 1996; NIOSH, 1993a; NIOSH, 1993b; NIOSH, 1996; Warshaw & Messite, 1996). As such, the following hypothesis was investigated:

Ha(6): The fewer the number of coworkers present while working with clients, the greater the likelihood and frequency of victimization by clients.

As for the number of coworkers present, none of the findings showed any significant relationship between the number of coworkers present and risk of victimization. Since the results do not show any differences in risk of victimization between employees who work with fewer coworkers and those who work with more coworkers, the null hypothesis fails to be rejected.

## Target Suitability

According to Nigro and Waugh (1996), trained employees in the area of violence prevention may also make the workplace environment a safer place. As such, the following hypotheses were investigated:

Ha(7): The more violence or crisis prevention training an employee has, the lower the likelihood and frequency of victimization by clients.

Ha(8): The more formal education an employee has, the lower the likelihood and frequency of victimization by clients.

Ha(9): The more job experience an employee has, the lower the likelihood and frequency of victimization by clients.

While it was initially expected that the findings would show that greater amounts of training would decrease one's risk of victimization, this was not the case. Rather, having more training appeared to increase one's probability of experiencing verbal abuse and physical victimization. Additionally, it was expected that the more educated employees would also experience less victimization. However, education seemed to have very little impact across the victimization models. Keeping in line with training and education, it was also expected that the more experienced employees would also experience less victimization. However, as with training and education, the expected findings were not supported. Rather, the more experienced employees experienced more victimization during their career as compared to those who had less experience. While it was initially expected that training, education, and experience would have a negative impact on victimization, the qualitative interviews also provided a different viewpoint. Some of the interviewees stated that while training and education benefits the employee as far as safety is concerned, it also increases awareness of victimization. As such, it appears that employees who were more aware of the violence were more apt to report such acts, versus those who were not as aware and who did not report victimization. Furthermore, one of the reasons that employees may not report the victimization is because they do not recognize it as violence. In addition, those employees with more training, education, and experience may also have more contact with more difficult clients, which may impact the likelihood of experiencing victimization. Therefore, based on the overall findings, it does not appear that there is support for alternative hypothesis #7, #8, or #9.

According to the literature, carrying drugs or having access to drugs, and working particular hours or shifts (i.e., late at night or during early morning) have been associated with an increased risk of victimization (LaMar et al., 1998; Nigro & Waugh, 1996; NIOSH, 1993a; NIOSH, 1993b; NIOSH, 1996; Warshaw & Messite, 1996). This suggests the following hypotheses:

Ha(10): Employees who have access to or carry narcotics while working are more likely and more often victimized by clients than those who do not.

Ha(11): Employees working more hours per week and those working late at night or during the early morning are more likely and more often victimized by clients than those who do not.

Based on the literature, it was expected that employees who had access to or carried drugs would experience greater victimization. The findings did not support this view. Only verbal victimization was higher for those employees who had access to or carried drugs. Thus, the quantitative findings provide weak support at best for alternative hypothesis #10.

As for the number of hours worked per week, there was a significant relationship apparent to victimization. The findings showed that the more hours an employee worked per week, the greater the probability of experiencing verbal abuse, threats, and physical victimization. In addition, as the literature suggested, working during the evening or at night also increased one's risk of victimization. The findings showed that those working during the day experienced less verbal abuse, threats, and physical victimization. Based on these findings, there is strong support for alternative hypothesis #11. Therefore, the null hypothesis is rejected, as there were significant differences among employees who worked during the day as compared to those who worked during the evening or at night.

Last, while demographic characteristics have been found to be statistically significant in victimization research, domain-specific research utilizing routine activities has found that demographic variables (e.g., gender, age) are less significant once routine activities variables are introduced (Lynch, 1987). Based on previous research (not restricted to the work domain), age and gender have been shown to have a relationship with risk of victimization (Lynch, 1987). As such, the following hypothesis was analyzed:

> Ha(12): The routine activities of employees play a
> greater role in the likelihood and frequency of
> victimization than do the demographic
> characteristics of employees.

Based on the literature, it was expected that males and younger employees would be more likely to experience victimization. The findings of this study provided weak to moderate support for this view. Males were more likely to experience verbal abuse and threats as compared to females. As for age, only one model showed a significant relationship. The findings showed that younger employees were more likely to experience threats as compared to older employees.

While not a traditional demographic variable, working style was also used as a measure of target suitability. The findings suggested that those who were more firm or assertive with their clients had a greater likelihood of experiencing victimization. For example, employees with a more assertive or firm demeanor experienced more threats and physical victimization in the past year as compared to employees who had a more relaxed or laid back demeanor.

Based on the findings, there was some support for the demographic variables. However, the employee's style and gender were stronger indicators as compared to the age of the employee. Furthermore, it appeared that the routine activities variables played a greater role overall in determining the likelihood and frequency of victimization. Working style seemed to have more of an impact than gender and age. This supports previous findings that demographic variables are less important when routine activities variables are introduced (Lynch, 1987). Therefore, there was support for hypothesis #12 and the null hypothesis was rejected.

## Descriptive Findings

Other variables were also measured in order to provide descriptive data, which revealed some interesting information about workplace violence in the field of mental health. The variables included were as follows: reporting procedures (PROCEDURES), reporting practices (PRACTICES), to whom violence is reported (SUPERVISOR, COWORKER, POLICE, FRIEND), whether or not a weapon was used in the commission of the act (WEAPON), and how violence is defined in the workplace (VERBAL ABUSE, THREATS OF HARM, PUSHING, HITTING, KICKING, BITING, PUNCHING, SLAPPING, CHOKING, SPITTING, THROWING OBJECTS, ROBBERY, RAPE, and SEXUAL ASSAULT). See Table 14.

The first variable examined reporting procedures (PROCEDURES). PROCEDURES was coded as either a zero or a one. If formal reporting procedures did not exist at the respondent's place of employment, the variable was coded as a zero. If formal reporting procedures did exist, the variable was coded as a one. The mean score for PROCEDURES was .92, indicating that 92% of those surveyed had formal reporting procedures at their place of employment.

Table 14: Other Descriptive Information

| Variable | Mean | SD | N |
|---|---|---|---|
| PROCEDURES | .92 | .28 | 423 |
| PRACTICES | .73 | .44 | 449 |
| SUPERVISOR | .65 | .48 | 449 |
| COWORKER | .53 | .50 | 449 |
| POLICE | .05 | .21 | 449 |
| FRIEND | .21 | .41 | 449 |
| WEAPON | .16 | .37 | 449 |
| VERBAL ABUSE | .55 | .50 | 449 |
| THREATS | .84 | .37 | 449 |
| PUSHING | .94 | .23 | 449 |
| HITTING | .97 | .16 | 449 |
| KICKING | .97 | .18 | 449 |
| BITING | .98 | .15 | 449 |
| PUNCHING | .99 | .11 | 449 |
| SLAPPING | .96 | .19 | 449 |
| CHOKING | .98 | .12 | 449 |
| SPITTING | .86 | .35 | 449 |
| THROWING OBJECTS | .98 | .52 | 449 |
| ROBBERY | .87 | .33 | 449 |
| RAPE | .99 | .09 | 449 |
| SEXUAL ASSAULT | .99 | .09 | 449 |

The next variable addressed the reporting practices of employees (PRACTICES), as well as to whom the violence is generally reported (SUPERVISOR, COWORKER, POLICE, FRIEND). Reporting practices were included to see if incidences of violence were primarily reported within the facility, to other agencies (such as the police), or not reported at all. The literature has indicated that reporting procedures are not uniform across employers (Peek-Asa et al., 1998).

PRACTICES was coded as either a zero or a one. If employees did not report the victimization, the variable was coded as a zero. If they reported the victimization, the variables was coded as a one. The mean score was .73, which indicates that 73% of those surveyed reported the victimization.

The next set of variables identified to whom the violence was reported. SUPERVISOR, COWORKER, POLICE, FRIEND were all coded as either a zero or a one. The mean score for SUPERVISOR was .65, which indicates that 65% of those surveyed reported the act to their supervisor. The mean score for COWORKER was .53, indicating that 53% of the respondents reported the act to another coworker. The mean score for POLICE was .05, which suggests that only 5% of the respondents reported their victimization to the police. The mean score for FRIEND was .21, indicating that 21% of those surveyed reported the victimization to a friend or family member. This is consistent with the literature, which states that this field has generally shown higher rates of victimization in victimization surveys as compared to police reports (Peek-Asa et al., 1998; Warchol, 1998). Thus, studies conducted using police reports as their primary source of information may greatly under represent the amount of victimization occurring in certain occupations, like the field of mental health.

The next variable refers to whether or not a weapon was used in the commission of the act (WEAPON). The variable was coded as either a zero or a one. If no weapon was used, the variable was coded as a zero. If a weapon was used to carry out the act, the variable was coded as a one. The mean score was .16, indicating that 16% of those surveyed stated that a weapon was used during the victimization. The types of weapons or objects used in the commission of the act varied. They included medication containers, screwdrivers, lamps, combs, television remotes, radios, umbrellas, books, vacuums, pictures on walls, toys, clothes, shoes, keys, jewelry, food trays, cups, rocks, knifes, forks, canes, pens, pool sticks, towel bars, hammers, ashtrays, guns, bow and arrows, lit cigarettes, brooms, and furniture.

The last set of variables look at how workplace violence is defined within the field of mental health. How one defines violence in the workplace is an important issue, as it differs across industries (Capozzoli & McVey, 1996; Nigro & Waugh, 1996; Warshaw & Messite, 1996). A question on the survey asked mental health workers what they considered to be violence in the workplace, and the acts were coded as either a zero or a one. If the act was not considered workplace violence, it was coded as a zero. If the act was considered workplace violence, it was coded as a one. The following acts were included on the survey and are listed with their mean score in parentheses: VERBAL ABUSE (.55), THREATS OF HARM (.84), PUSHING

(.94), HITTING (.97), KICKING (.97), BITING (.98), PUNCHING
(.99), SLAPPING (.96), CHOKING (.98), SPITTING (.86),
THROWING OBJECTS (.98), ROBBERY (.87), RAPE (.99), and
SEXUAL ASSAULT (.99). While only approximately half of those
surveyed considered verbal abuse or swearing to be violence,
approximately 95% of those surveyed considered various physical acts
to be violent (i.e., pushing, hitting, kicking, biting, punching, slapping,
choking, throwing objects, rape, and other types of sexual assault). The
only exceptions were spitting and robbery. Approximately 86% - 87%
of those surveyed considered spitting and robbery to be acts of
workplace violence. As for threats of physical harm, approximately
84% considered it to be violence.

## Summary

The quantitative findings showed that several of the independent
variables, used as measures of the three elements of routine activities
theory, had significant impact on the dependent variables. Upon
examining the first set of independent variables, which provided
measures of exposure to potential offenders, perceptions of danger
provided the strongest support for the alternative hypotheses. That is to
say that those employees who viewed more of their weekly client
contacts as dangerous were more likely to experience victimization.
Type of mental disorder, number of weekly client contacts, and setting
provided weak or no support for the alternative hypotheses, in that the
variables did not have a significant impact on victimization.

It also should be noted that the findings from the qualitative
interviews were consistent with the quantitative findings regarding type
of mental disorder. While some of those interviewed did feel that
schizophrenia and other psychotic disorders may put one at an
increased risk of violence, many stated that other factors, not
necessarily disorder type, have more of an effect on risk. For example,
clients who are decompensating, who are not taking their medications
properly, have no social support, have a history of prior abuse, and/or
have issues with drugs and alcohol may pose an increased risk.

For the next set of variables, which provided measures of
guardianship, the type of facility provided the strongest support, in that
those working in crisis facilities were more likely to experience

victimization than those working in residential and/or nonresidential facilities. The number of coworkers present provided little or no support for the alternative hypothesis, in that the variable did not have a significant impact on victimization.

For the next set of independent variables, which provided measures of target suitability, the number of hours and time of day worked per week, gender, and style provided strong support for the alternative hypotheses. This was consistent with the literature that states working evening or night shifts is associated with an increased risk of victimization (LaMar et al., 1998; Nigro & Waugh, 1996; NIOSH, 1993a, NIOSH, 1993b, NIOSH, 1996, Warshaw & Messite, 1996). The literature also supports the findings concerning gender, which states males are more likely to be victimized than females. The only exception is rape and other types of sexual assault, in which females make up the majority of victims (Warchol, 1998). Training, education, experience, drugs and age provided weak or no support for the alternative hypotheses, in that the variables did not have a significant impact on victimization.

However, the qualitative interviews conducted exemplified a different viewpoint concerning education, training, and experience. Specifically, while education and training were seen as important in respect to workplace safety, they also appear to heighten the awareness of the employee. It is this heightened awareness that many believed keeps workers safe. However, it also seems that this awareness may contribute to a positive relationship between experience and victimization, as well as between education and victimization. In other words, it may be that employees who are more aware of potential victimization, may also be more likely to recognize and report such victimization. It would also make sense that this same relationship would be found with regard to experience, as the more experience one has, the more likely one would be to recognize and report victimization as well.

The descriptive data showed some interesting information about violence in the workplace in the field of mental health. First, the data revealed that most employees (92%) reported having formal reporting procedures at their place of employment. The data also showed that the majority of the employees reported any incidences of violence to their supervisor. Generally speaking, most reporting occurred within the facility. Seventy-three percent of those surveyed reported the victimization, with 65% of those surveyed reporting the act to their supervisor and only 5% reporting to the police. These findings were consistent with the literature, which states that this field has generally shown higher rates of victimization in victimization surveys as compared to police reports (Peek-Asa et al., 1998; Warchol, 1998). As such, using police reports as the primary source of information may greatly underrepresent the amount of victimization occurring in certain occupations, like the field of mental health. Finally, most of the respondents considered physical acts of violence to be workplace violence. Physical acts considered violence included pushing, hitting, kicking, biting, punching, slapping, choking, spitting, throwing objects, robbery, rape, and sexual assault. Eighty-four percent considered threats of harm to be violence, and 55% considered verbal abuse to be workplace violence.

# CHAPTER VI

# Practical Implications

Based on this study, some of the findings provided strong support for routine activities theory, as well as providing rich data about violence in the field of mental health. In addition, there are several policy or practical implications that may be drawn from this study.

## Exposure to Potential Offenders

Based on the literature (Arango et al., 1999; Link et al., 1992; Modestin & Ammann, 1996; Taylor et al., 1998; Wessely et al., 1994), it was expected that those employees working with clients suffering from more acute mental illness would experience greater victimization. Studies have shown that certain types of mentally ill patients or clients are more prone to violence than others (Arango et al., 1999; Link et al., 1992; Modestin & Ammann, 1996; Taylor et al., 1998; Wessely et al., 1994), and higher rates of violence have also been associated with more acute mental illness (Modestin & Ammann, 1996). For example, Wessely et al. (1994) studied 538 schizophrenics and found that these men and women posed a greater risk for committing violent acts than did those in the comparison groups (i.e., persons with other psychiatric diagnoses). Overall, these findings suggested that schizophrenic patients, compared to those with other psychiatric conditions, have an increased risk of offending. In another study, Bartels et al. (1991) found that that those who were more hostile were more likely to abuse drugs and alcohol. Fifty-nine percent of the patients rated as violent in that study were found to have a substance abuse problem. With this research in mind, it was expected in the current research that clients having dual diagnoses or schizophrenia would be more apt to be violent than those with other types of diagnoses.

However, this was simply not the case. In this study, a number of variables were used to measure exposure to potential offenders, and few were found to have an impact on victimization. First, the findings showed that there was a weak relationship between working with the more severely mentally ill and victimization. Approximately 60% of the respondents reported working regularly with schizophrenics. While working regularly with schizophrenics did have a positive impact in some of the models that examined verbal victimization, there was a negative impact in some of the linear models that examined threats and physical victimization. This actually suggests that, among those who were threatened or physically victimized, working regularly with schizophrenics decreased one's frequency of encountering threats or physical acts of violence.

As for employees working regularly with substance abusers, somewhat similar findings were uncovered. Approximately 37% of the respondents reported working regularly with clients with substance-related problems. Doing so was found to have a negative impact in the linear models examining verbal victimization and threats, which suggests that, among those verbally victimized and threatened, those working regularly with substance abusers experienced a lower frequency of verbal abuse and threats. No significance was found within any of the models examining physical acts of violence. Although the findings of this study contradicted some of the existing research, it also appears that there is controversy in the literature with respect to the actual risk posed by the mentally ill (Baron & Neuman, 1996; Capozzoli & McVey, 1996; Labig, 1995; Monahan & Arnold, 1996; Nigro & Waugh, 1996; Warshaw & Messite, 1996). Some recent studies have stated that the mentally ill pose no more of a threat than the general population.

Similar to the research discussed above, mixed views were also apparent among those employees interviewed for this study. About half of the interviewees associated schizophrenia and other psychotic disorders with an increased risk of violence, which is consistent with much of the literature (Arango et al., 1999; Link et al., 1992; Modestin & Ammann, 1996; Taylor et al., 1998; Wessely et al., 1994). About one-third of those interviewed believed that there was an increased risk of violence among those with substance-related disorders. In most cases, interviewees believed that the risk was higher among those clients with comorbidity or a dual diagnosis, which was also consistent with the literature (Bartels et al., 1991; Swanson et al., 1990). However, many of the interviewees suggested that specific diagnoses were not necessarily reflective of a greater propensity towards violence. Rather, they believed other factors may play a greater role in contributing to violence. For example, clients who are decompensating, are not taking their medications properly, have no social support, and have a history of prior abuse may also be at an increased risk of violent offending. As such, the weight of the quantitative and qualitative evidence would suggest that working with clients with more severe mental illness does not necessarily increase one's risk of victimization, but rather more specific client and situational based factors may be more important. If this is true, these factors might also raise perceptions of danger on the part of employees.

As for these perceptions of danger on the part of mental health workers, it was expected that those who perceived greater danger among their weekly client contacts would experience greater victimization. As expected, the quantitative findings showed that those who perceived greater danger were more likely and more often victimized. While the average employee viewed approximately three of their weekly client contacts as dangerous, about half of those surveyed indicated that none or only one of their weekly client contacts posed a threat of danger. Overall, perceived danger had a positive impact on all types of victimization, including verbal, threats, and physical victimization. Specifically, the findings suggest that employees who perceive more of their weekly client contacts as dangerous experience a greater frequency of verbal abuse, and they are both more likely to experience, and experience a greater frequency of, threats and physical victimization. Therefore, the findings indicate that there is a positive relationship between perceptions of dangerous client contacts and victimization. These findings also agree with past literature (Lynch, 1987; Wooldredge et al., 1992), which suggests that there is a relationship between perceived dangerousness of clients and victimization.

However, it should also be noted that there are other plausible explanations for the strong and consistent relationship between perceived dangerousness and victimization. First, it could be that employees who have experienced greater victimization perceive their clients to be more dangerous because of the previous victimization experiences (with the same client or other clients). Thus, it may be that their previous victimization experiences are affecting their perceptions of danger. Second, both perceived dangerousness and victimization might also be influenced by how employees relate with their clients. Thus, how they interact with clients on a regular basis may lead to increased perceptions of danger and victimization. Finally, it may be that experienced mental health workers are good at assessing risk and violence potential, which may account for the higher levels of victimization experienced.

Based on the literature, it also was expected that as the number of weekly client contacts increased, so would victimization. The literature has indicated that working with capricious individuals (i.e., in health care, social service, or criminal justice settings) plays a role in workplace victimization (LaMar et al., 1998; Nigro & Waugh, 1996; NIOSH, 1993a, NIOSH, 1993b; NIOSH, 1996; Warshaw & Messite, 1996).

A review of the quantitative findings showed that greater numbers of client contacts had a positive impact in some of the models examining verbal victimization, but this variable did not have any significant impact in the models examining threats or physical victimization. The average number of weekly client contacts among respondents was 25. The positive impact between weekly client contacts and verbal abuse suggests that as the number of client contacts on a weekly basis increases, so does the likelihood of experiencing verbal abuse.

Similarly, the qualitative interviews revealed that most of the interviewees characterized verbal abuse and swearing as occurring on a more frequent basis, as compared to other types of victimization. However, the overall findings suggest that there is only weak support for the relationship between the number of weekly client contacts and violent victimization.

Finally, based on the literature, it was expected that employees working in urban areas would experience more victimization. Studies have shown that working in crime-prone areas, such as urban environments, plays a role in workplace victimization (LaMar et al., 1998; Nigro & Waugh, 1996; NIOSH, 1993a, NIOSH, 1993b; NIOSH, 1996; Warshaw & Messite, 1996). However, this was not the case in the current research, as working in an urban environment did not have a strong or consistent impact on victimization. Overall, 41% of the employees reported working in an urban area. This had a significant, positive impact in only one of the verbal models, suggesting that employees working in an urban environment had a greater likelihood of experiencing verbal abuse. No significant impact was found in the other models examining threats and physical victimization. It appears that there is very weak support for the relationship between working in urban areas and victimization. Furthermore, working in a suburban environment also had little impact across the victimization models.

Overall, while this study attempted to provide a further examination of the importance of exposure to potential offenders, the findings did not provide strong evidence of support for this element. While this study attempted to better operationalize exposure to potential offenders in order to produce a sounder model, and found that greater perceived danger was positively related to victimization, it does not appear that the overall objective was fully satisfied. It would seem that additional testing must be conducted, with an emphasis on further operationalization of this element. Specifically, future research should focus on the client and situational based factors that may produce a "dangerous" encounter for mental health employees, and also consider how employees handle or deal with these particular factors.

## Guardianship

A variety of variables also were used to measure guardianship. Based on the findings, several were found to have an impact on victimization. As for the first variable, number of coworkers present, studies have shown that employees who work alone or in small groups are more likely to experience victimization (LaMar et al., 1998; Nigro & Waugh, 1996; NIOSH, 1993a; NIOSH, 1993b; NIOSH, 1996; Warshaw & Messite, 1996). However, the quantitative findings did not support this conclusion, as no significance was found for this variable. According to the respondents, the average number of coworkers present during client contacts was five, with approximately 25% reporting that they typically worked alone. None of the models produced any significant relationship between number of coworkers present and risk of victimization.

For the next variable, facility type, the literature has indicated that the risk of victimization varies according to the environment (Warshaw and Messite, 1996). For example, although those who are hospitalized tend to be more ill, they generally are also receiving more supervision, medication, care, and support as compared to those who are living in the community. Upon considering the facility in which one is employed, it was expected that those working in crisis facilities would be more likely to experience victimization than those working in residential and nonresidential facilities. Based on the quantitative findings, facility type was found to have a significant impact on victimization.

Thirty-six percent of those surveyed reported working in a nonresidential facility. Working in a nonresidential facility was found to have a negative impact in some of the victimization models examining threats of harm. This suggests that those working in nonresidential facilities have a lower likelihood of experiencing threats than those working in crisis facilities. No significance was found among the models examining verbal abuse or physical victimization.

Thirty-five percent of those surveyed worked in residential facilities. A significant negative impact was found in some of the models examining threats and physical victimization. This suggests that employees working in residential facilities have a lower likelihood of experiencing threats or physical victimization than those working in crisis facilities. Based on these findings, there is at least moderate support for the conclusion that employees working in crisis facilities have a greater likelihood of being victimized by clients than those working in nonresidential and residential facilities.

According to those interviewed, perceptions of the impact of type of facility in which one works on victimization risk appeared to vary. For example, some interviewees believed that consumers who are currently in a residential or inpatient setting are more likely to act out than consumers in other types of settings. Those interviewed attributed this to the fact that consumers in residential and inpatient settings are generally sicker and more unstable than those who are living in the community, which is why they are receiving more intensive services. In addition, mental health workers spend more time with clients in residential and inpatient settings, which may allow more opportunities for violence to occur.

However, some interviewees believed that working with clients in the community, in crisis situations, could pose a greater risk. This may be due to the fact that when consumers are in crisis, generally they are unstable, volatile, and decompensating, which may increase their propensity towards violence. There is also less structure when clients are living in the community, which can be an added stressor when the consumer is in crisis. Additionally, there is also less supervision of medications, which may increase the chance for decomposition.

Another setting where clients were viewed to possibly pose an increased risk included outpatient settings, especially involving those services that included home visits. In outpatient settings, it appears more difficult to control the environment. The usual precautions that might normally be taken may be difficult in an outpatient setting, thereby increasing one's risk.

Overall, strong support was found for facility type, which supports this routine activity element. No support was found for number of coworkers typically present. Additionally, level of guardianship appears to provide a better predictor of victimization as compared to exposure to potential offenders.

## Target Suitability

Finally, a variety of variables were used to measure target suitability. Based on the findings, several were found to have an impact on victimization. As for training, education, and experience, it was expected that all three would have a significant, negative impact on victimization. According to Nigro and Waugh (1996), training employees in the area of violence prevention should result in a safer workplace environment, and subsequently, a lesser frequency of victimization. However, this was not the case in this study. The findings indicated that all three variables had a positive, significant impact in many of the victimization models. This suggests that the more training, education, and experience an employee has, the greater the likelihood and frequency of experiencing victimization.

However, while it was initially expected that training, education, and experience would have a negative impact on victimization, the qualitative interviews hinted at a different viewpoint. Some of the interviewees stated that while training benefits the employee as far as safety is concerned, it also increases awareness of victimization. As such, it seems that employees who were more aware of the violence may have been more apt to report such acts in this study, versus those who were not as aware. It is also this heightened awareness that many believed kept workers safe. Furthermore, one of the reasons that employees may not formally report victimization is because they might not recognize it as violence. In addition, it should also be considered that those employees with more training, education, and experience might be assigned more high-risk clients to work with on a regular basis. As a result, those employees may experience greater exposure to possible victimization. Additionally, those employees who work with high-risk clients might also seek out more training and education to assist them with their more difficult clients. While the overall findings were different from the expected outcomes, all the variables were found to have a significant impact on victimization. The qualitative interviews also suggest that the importance of training, education, and experience should not be ignored.

As for training, the average amount of violence or crisis prevention training employees reported experiencing in the past year was 6 _ hours. This variable had a positive impact in some of the models examining verbal abuse and physical victimization. This suggests that those employees with more training have a greater likelihood and frequency of verbal abuse and physical victimization. As for threats, none of the coefficients for training were significant. However, this is not to say that training causes victimization, but rather that trained employees may be more aware of the potential for violence or handle more difficult cases.

As for education, the average employee had a Bachelor's degree. This variable was found to have a positive impact in only one model, examining verbal victimization. Thus, those with more education were found to have a greater likelihood of experiencing verbal abuse in their career. There was no significance found in any of the models examining threats or physical victimization. Again, as with training, it might also be that the more educated employees deal with difficult clients and have heightened awareness.

As for experience, the average worker had approximately nine years of experience in the field of mental health. While experience did not have a significant impact on more recent victimization, this variable was found to have a positive impact in the logistic regression models examining career victimization, including those for verbal abuse, threats, and physical victimization. This suggests that those employees with more experience have a greater likelihood of experiencing verbal abuse, threats, and physical victimization. One could draw the conclusion that has with training and experience, those with more experience may also be more inclined to handle the difficult cases and would most certainly be aware of and able to recognize violence.

As for the variable, drugs, the literature suggests that carrying drugs or having access to drugs is associated with an increased risk of victimization (LaMar et al., 1998; Nigro & Waugh, 1996; NIOSH, 1993a; NIOSH, 1993b; NIOSH, 1996; Warshaw & Messite, 1996). However, the quantitative findings did not provide much support for this conclusion. On average, 37% of those surveyed reported having access to or carrying drugs while working. This was found to have a positive impact in only one of the victimization models, which examined verbal abuse. Specifically, the findings suggested that, among those verbally victimized in the past 12 months, the frequency of victimization was higher for those employees who had access to or carried drugs. Since there was no significant impact found in the other victimization models, only very weak support was found for the importance of this variable.

For the next two variables, the literature has suggested that working particular hours or shifts (i.e., late at night or during the early morning) is associated with an increased risk of victimization (LaMar et al., 1998; Nigro & Waugh, 1996; NIOSH, 1993a; NIOSH, 1993b; NIOSH, 1996; Warshaw & Messite, 1996). As for the number of hours worked per week and time of day worked, a significant impact was found within some of the victimization models. On average, respondents worked approximately 39 hours per week. This variable was found to be significant in six of the models examining verbal abuse, threats, and physical victimization. Hours worked had a positive impact on the dependent variables, suggesting that the more hours worked per week by employees, the greater the likelihood that they would experience some type of victimization, including verbal abuse, threats, and physical victimization.

As for the time of day, 63% of those surveyed reported typically working during the day shift. This variable had a significant, negative impact in some of the models examining verbal abuse, threats, and physical victimization. This indicates that employees working an evening or night shift have a greater likelihood of experiencing verbal abuse, threats, and physical victimization, as compared to those who work during the day. Based on these overall findings, there is strong support that these variables have an impact on victimization.

Last, while demographic characteristics have been found to be statistically significant in victimization research, domain-specific research utilizing routine activities theory has found that demographic variables (e.g., gender, age) are less significant once routine activities variables are introduced (Lynch, 1987). Based on previous research (not restricted to the work domain), age and gender have been shown to have a relationship with risk of victimization (Lynch, 1987). In this study, it was expected that the routine activities of employees would play a greater role in the likelihood and frequency of victimization than would the demographic characteristics of employees. The quantitative findings showed that age and gender were found to have a significant impact in few of the victimization models. The average age of the employee in this study was 39 _ years old, with 73% of those surveyed being female. Age was found to have a negative impact in only one of the models, examining threats. This suggests that younger employees are more likely to experience threats. No significance was found in any of the models examining verbal abuse or physical victimization.

As for gender, there was a significant, negative impact in the models examining verbal abuse and threats. This suggests that males are more likely to experience verbal abuse and threats than females. No significance was found in any of the physical victimization models. The literature supports these findings concerning gender, also showing that males are more likely to be victimized than females.

While not a traditional demographic variable, working style was also used as a measure of target suitability. The respondents were asked to characterize their style on a scale of zero to ten (i.e., 0=very relaxed/laid back; 10=very assertive/firm). The mean respondent score was 5.14, indicating that the average employee was in the middle of the two ends of the spectrum. The findings indicated that this variable had a fairly consistent, positive impact in the models examining verbal abuse, threats, and physical victimization. This positive effect suggests that those who are more firm or assertive with their clients have a greater likelihood of experiencing verbal abuse and threats, and among those physically victimized, experience a greater frequency of physical victimization.

Based on the findings, there is moderate support for the demographic variables. Gender was a stronger predictor as compared to age. However, it appears that the routine activities variables played a greater role overall in determining the likelihood and frequency of victimization. In particular, working style seemed to have a consistent, positive impact. Furthermore, it appears that there is moderate support for the impact of the variables measuring the concept of target suitability.

Overall, the quantitative findings showed that several of the independent variables, used as measures of the three elements of routine activities theory, had a significant impact in the victimization models. Of all three of the elements, exposure to potential offenders appeared to receive the weakest support compared to the other two elements. Perceptions of danger and, to a lesser extent, location, received the strongest support, while type of mental disorder and number of weekly client contacts received little or no support. For the element of guardianship, type of facility received the strongest support, in contrast to the number of coworkers present. As for the element of target suitability, the number of hours worked per week, time of day worked, training, education, experience, gender, and style all received some or strong support. Drugs and age received little or no support.

## Descriptive Data

According to the findings, 85% of the respondents reported being verbally abused at some point in their career. Fifty-five percent had experienced threats, and 52% had experienced physical victimization. When asked to indicate any violence they had experienced in the past year, the percentage of violence reported dropped. For example, only 75% of the respondents reported being verbally abused, only 40% had been threatened, and only 35% experienced physical victimization in the past year. As for formally reporting the violence, when respondents were asked about procedures and practices at their workplace, the findings were interesting. While 92% of those surveyed reported the existence of formal procedures at their place of employment, only 73% of those surveyed had used them.

The qualitative interviews suggested that reporting of incidences would be higher than what was revealed in the survey data. All of those interviewed stated that any violence they experienced was reported.  As for formal reporting procedures, 87% of those interviewed indicated that they were aware of reporting procedures within their agency, which is comparable to the quantitative findings. However, the fact that not all employees report all incidences was also apparent in the qualitative findings, as some interviewees believed that there was underreporting among staff.  They attributed this to fear of liability, not wanting to get the client in trouble, as well as either not wanting to or forgetting to fill out the paperwork.

As to whom the victimization was reported, the answers varied. The literature has indicated that this field has generally shown higher rates of victimization in victimization surveys as compared to police reports (Peek-Asa et al., 1998; Warchol, 1998).  For example, Warchol (1998) found that health professionals reported less than half of all nonfatal victimizations to the police, as it generally was reported to another official.  Thus, studies conducted using police reports as their primary source of information may greatly under-represent the amount of victimization occurring in certain occupations like the field of mental health.

The quantitative findings were consistent with the literature. Sixty-five percent of those surveyed reported the act to their supervisor, 53% of the respondents reported the act to another coworker, only 5% reported to the police, and 21% reported the victimization to a friend or family member.  As the literature suggests, it is interesting to note the small percentage of victimization that is actually reported to the police.

The qualitative interviews were also consistent with the quantitative findings.  Some interviewees stated that reporting typically was done within the facility, and that reporting practices were not uniform across facilities.  One interviewee stated that there are formal procedures at all levels—state, county, and agency levels—which give direction on how to complete reports, such as unusual incident reports. From the interviews, it appeared that the unusual incident report forms filed with the county and regional Mental Health/Mental Retardation offices were the only identified uniform practice in the field.  Other than that, it appeared that reporting varied across facilities, subject to the internal incident reports.

As to whom the violence was reported, the reporting practices of the interviewees were similar to those from the survey.  Sixty-five percent of those interviewed stated that they reported the act to their supervisor, and 54% reported the act to another coworker. In general, the reporting of such acts was done internally, and the immediate supervisor was generally notified first. Less than 6% of those interviewed filed a report with the police. According to most of the interviewees, the police were not involved unless some type of physical act resulting in bodily harm or medical treatment had occurred, or if charges were to be filed. Most stated that they discussed the situation with their supervisor first, or simply did not take the threat serious enough to warrant calling the police. In other cases, the act may not be reported to the police, or even to the employer for that matter, because it is not recognized as workplace violence (NIOSH, 1996, Warshaw & Messite, 1996). However, reporting to the police appears to be based on perceptions of the individual worker as to how serious they view the situation. There did not appear to be any hard and fast rules.

As for the use of a weapon during the commission of an act, the quantitative findings suggested that weapons are not used frequently. The findings indicated that 16% of those surveyed stated that a weapon was used during the victimization. The types of weapons or objects used in the commission of the act included medication containers, screwdrivers, lamps, combs, television remotes, radios, umbrellas, books, vacuums, pictures on walls, toys, clothes, shoes, keys, jewelry, food trays, cups, rocks, knifes, forks, canes, pens, pool sticks, towel bars, hammers, ashtrays, guns, bow and arrows, lit cigarettes, brooms, and furniture. The qualitative interviews also did not suggest that weapons were used in many of the victimizations.

Last, how workplace violence is defined within the field of mental health was also addressed. This definition is an important issue, as it differs across industries (Capozzoli & McVey, 1996; Nigro & Waugh, 1996; Warshaw & Messite, 1996). How violence was defined varied, but most of the respondents viewed the following acts as violence: pushing, hitting, kicking, biting, punching, slapping, choking, spitting, throwing objects, robbery, rape, and sexual assault. With the exceptions of robbery and spitting, at least 94% of the respondents viewed those acts as violence. Approximately 86% - 87% of those surveyed considered spitting and robbery to be acts of workplace violence. It may be that the robbery percentage is lower because of differing definitions of what constitutes robbery. For example, some respondents may view robbery as simply theft and not as a violent crime. As for threats of harm, 84% of the respondents viewed them as violence. Verbal abuse was considered to be violence by 55% of those surveyed.

These findings are consistent with the qualitative data. According to the interviewees, what one employee considers violence might be considered by someone else as part of the job or simply an annoyance. For example, some interviewees believed that violence was more than just swearing or verbal abuse alone. Verbal threats appeared to be taken seriously by many of those interviewed, especially when a weapon or object was involved. However, some interviewees stated that the threats must also be accompanied by a means of carrying out the threat. Others interviewed viewed violence not as merely threats, but rather physical threats of assault. While not everyone considered acts such as verbal abuse, swearing, or threats of physical harm to be violence, all interviewees unanimously defined violence to include physical acts, which included behaviors such as pushing, hitting, kicking, biting, punching, slapping, choking, spitting, throwing objects, robbery, rape, and other types of sexual assault.

# Practical Applications: Where do we go from here?

Based on the findings of this study, it appears that certain measures should be taken to address the issue of workplace violence in the field of mental health. First, it would be helpful if there were uniform reporting practices across facilities. For example, facilities could have stronger guidelines in place as to when police should be involved. As for perceptions about the violent tendencies of the mentally ill, it would seem that the perceived frequency of violence in this field depends upon how that violence is defined. While it would be helpful to have a uniform definition of what constitutes violence, this may be difficult to achieve due to differing perceptions of victimization. For example, some employees consider verbal abuse to be violence, while others perceive it to be part of the job. In addition, while it seems efficient that a majority of reporting is done internally, facilities should continue to report to outside agencies (e.g., county and regional Mental Health/Mental Retardation) when it is warranted. The use of the unusual incident reports appears to address the issue of violence in the workplace.

Second, while the hypotheses regarding training, education, and experience were not directly supported, the overall findings of this study did indicate the importance of these factors. Continual training and education, as well as job experience, appear to keep workers safe through heightening their awareness about violence. In addition, it also appears that training, education, and experience may also play a role in the increased reporting of such incidences. This is due to the fact that employees are aware of it and recognize the acts as violence. Thus, employees are more apt to report such incidences. This increased reporting leads to a more accurate picture of violence in the field, and the information can be utilized to maintain worker safety.

Third, it would appear that based on the findings, more testing of the importance of exposure to potential offenders is warranted. In particular, the specific client and situational based factors that create "dangerous" encounters and increase victimization risk on the part of mental health workers merits further research attention. Additionally, more testing of routine activities theory should be conducted in the context of domain specific research (e.g., whether that be in the workplace, home, or school, as well as other occupations). Further domain specific research will lead to more information regarding victimization that occurs in specific places and involves particular activities. Furthermore, by narrowing the scope of inquiry in utilizing domain specific victimization models, the explanatory power of routine activities theory might be more fully realized.

Finally, it would seem that general beliefs that the mentally ill are dangerous are unwarranted. While this study's purpose was not to address the ongoing debate regarding the mentally ill and their propensity towards violence, it does appear after examining the data that further research attention is warranted. It would appear that media attention and myths within the community have created a false sense of fear with regard to the actual risk that the mentally ill pose. Most of the interviewees believed that with the exception of profanity or verbal abuse, violence in this field is not as common as people believe. Furthermore, there appear to be contradictions in the literature. Based on the quantitative findings of this study, it appears that even the more severe mentally ill are not as violent as many believe them to be. All of those interviewed stated that the mentally ill are no more violent than anyone else in the general population, which is consistent with the recent literature (Bower, 1998; Monahan & Arnold, 1996; Steadman et al., 1998). The apparent contradiction in the literature, coupled with the findings of this study, make it clear that more research is necessary overall or at least clarity on how we define violence. The quantitative findings showed that most employees did not consider their clients to be dangerous, which supports the interview data. One final note, during an interview one employee said regarding workplace violence, "Violence is part of the job because you are dealing with people in general and it is inherent in society, not just the mentally ill." It would seem that this point is not disputed.

# References

Anderson, C., & Stamper, M. (2001). Workplace violence. *RN, 64* (2), 71.

Appelbaum, P., Robbins, P., & Monahan, J. (2000). Violence and delusions: Data from the Macarthur violence risk assessment study. *American Journal of Psychiatry, 157* (4), 566(7).

Arango, C., Barba, A., Gonzalez-Salvador, T., & Ordonez, A. (1999). Violence in inpatients with schizophrenia: A prospective study. *Schizophrenia Bulletin, 25* (3), 493-503.

Arseneault, L., Moffitt, T., Caspi, A., Taylor, P., & Silva, P. (2000). Mental disorders and violence in a total birth cohort: Results from the Dunedin study. *Archives of General Psychiatry, 57* (10), 979.

Babbie, E. (1995). *The practice of social research* (7th ed.). Belmont, CA: Wadsworth Publishing Company.

Babbie, E. (1997). *Survey research methods* (2nd ed.). Belmont, CA: Wadsworth Publishing Company.

Bachman, R., & Paternoster, R. (1997). *Statistical methods for criminology and criminal justice.* New York: McGraw-Hill.

Baron, R., & Neuman, J. (1996). Workplace violence and workplace aggression: Evidence of their relative frequency and potential causes. *Aggressive Behavior, 22,* 161-173.

Bartels, J., Drake, R., Wallach, M., & Freeman, D. (1991). Characteristic hostility in schizophrenic outpatients. *Schizophrenia Bulletin, 17* (1), 163-171.

Bennett, R. (1991). Routine activities: A cross-national assessment of a criminological perspective. *Social Forces, 70* (1), 147-163.

Block, R., Felson, M., & Block, C. (1984). Crime victimization rates for incumbents of 246 occupations. *Sociology and Social Research, 69* (3), 442-451.

Bower, B. (1998). Study tracks violence among mentally ill. *Science News, 153* (20), 309.

Bryant, K., & Miller, J. (1997). Routine activity and labor market segmentation: An empirical test of a revised approach. *American Journal of Criminal Justice, 22* (1), 71-100.

Calabrese, K. (2000). Interpersonal conflict and sarcasm in the workplace. *Genetic, Social, and General Psychology Monographs, 126* (4), 459.

Cao, L, & Maume, D. (1993). Urbanization, inequality, lifestyles and robbery: A comprehensive model. *Sociological Focus, 26* (1), 11-26.

Capozzoli, T., & McVey, R. S. (1996). *Managing violence in the workplace.* Delray Beach, FL: St. Lucie Press.

Carroll, V. (1996). Violence in the workplace: We are the missing link. *American Journal of Nursing, 96* (12), 80(1).

Chamlin, M., & Cochran, J. (1994). Opportunity, motivation, and assaults on police: A bivariate arima analysis. *American Journal of Criminal Justice, 19 (1),* 1-19.

Cohen, L., & Cantor, D. (1980). The determinants of larceny: An empirical and theoretical study. *Journal of Research in Crime and Delinquency,* July 1980, 140-159.

Cohen, L., Cantor, D., & Kluegel, J. (1981). Robbery victimization in the u.s.: An analysis of a nonrandom event. *Social Science Quarterly, 62* (4), 644-657.

Cohen, L., & Felson, M. (1979). Social change and crime rate trends: A routine activity approach. *American Sociological Review, 44* (August), 588-608.

Cohen, L., Kluegel, J., & Land, K. (1981a). Social inequality and predatory criminal victimization: An exposition and test of a formal theory. *American Sociological Review, 46,* 505-524.

Collins, J., Cox, B., & Langan, P. (1987). Job activities and personal crime victimization: Implications for theory. *Social Science Research, 16,* 345-360.

Creswell, J. (1994). *Research design: Qualitative and quantitative approaches.* Thousand Oaks, CA: Sage Publications, Inc.

DeCoster, S., Estes, S., & Mueller, C. (1999). Routine activities and sexual harassment in the workplace. *Work and Occupations, 26* (1), 21(29).

Ehrhardt-Mustaine, E. (1999). A routine activity theory explanation for women's stalking victimizations. *Violence Against Women, 5* (1), 43(20).

Ehrhardt-Mustaine, E., & Tewksbury, R. (1997). The risk of victimization in the workplace for men and women: An analysis using routine activities/lifestyle theory. *Humanity and Society, 21* (1), 17-38.

Ehrhardt-Mustaine, E., & Tewksbury, R. (1997a). Obstacles in the assessment of routine activity theory. *Social Pathology, 3* (3), 177-194.

Ehrhardt-Mustaine, E., & Tewksbury, R. (1998). Predicting risks of larceny theft victimization: A routine activity analysis using refined lifestyle measures. *Criminology, 36* (4), 829-857.

Eronen, M., Tiihonen, J., & Hakola, P. (1996). Schizophrenia and homicidal behavior. *Schizophrenia Bulletin 22,* 83-89.

Felson, M. (1996). Preventing retail theft: An application of environmental criminology. *Security Journal, 7,* 71-75.

Felson, M. (1987). Routine activities and crime prevention in the developing metropolis. *Criminology, 25* (4), 911-931.

Felson, M., & Cohen, L. (1980). Human ecology and crime: A routine activity approach. *Human Ecology, 8* (4), 389-406.

Finch, J. (1998). Social undermining, support satisfaction, and affect: A domain-specific lagged effects model. *Journal of Personality, 66* (3), 315(20).

Finkelhor, D., & Asdigian, N. (1996). Risk factors for youth victimization: Beyond a lifestyles/routine activities theory approach. *Violence and Victims, 11* (1), p. 3-19.

Finkelhor, D., & Ormrod, R. (1999). Reporting crimes against juveniles. *Juvenile Justice Bulletin,* November (NCJ178887).

Fowler, F. (1993). *Survey Research Methods* (2nd ed.). Newbury Park, CA: Sage Publications, Inc.

Garofalo, J., Siegel, L., & Laub, J. (1987). School-related victimizations among adolescents: An analysis of national crime survey (NCS) narratives. *Journal of Quantitative Criminology, 3* (4), 321-338.

George, R., & Thomas, G. (2000). Victimization among middle and high school students: A multilevel analysis. *The High School Journal, 84* (1), 48-57.

Harris, D., & Benson, M. (1998). Nursing home theft: The hidden problem. *Journal of Aging Studies, 12* (1), 57(11).

Hashemi, L., & Webster, B. S. (1998). Non-fatal workplace violence workers' compensation claims (1993-1996*). Journal of Occupational and Environmental Medicine, 40* (6), 561(7).

Hawley, A. (1950). *Human ecology.* New York: The Ronald Press Company.

Hindelang, M. (1976). *Criminal victimization in eight American cities.* Cambridge, MA: Ballinger.

Hindelang, M., Gottfredson, M., & Garofalo, J. (1978). *Victims of Personal Crime: An Empirical Foundation For a Theory of Personal Victimization.* Cambridge, MA: Ballinger Publishing Company.

Hlebovy, D. (2000). Violence in the workplace. *Nephrology Nursing Journal,* *27* (6), 631.

Hoag-Apel, C. M. (1998). Violence in the emergency department. *Nursing Management, 29* (7), 60(2).

Hodgins, S. (1992). Mental disorder, intellectual deficiency, and crime: Evidence from a birth cohort. *Archives of General Psychiatry, 49,* 476-483.

Hodgins, S., Mednick, S., Brennan, P., Schulsinger, F., & Engberg, M. (1996). Mental disorder and crime: Evidence from a danish birth cohort. *Archives of General Psychiatry,* 53, 489-496.

Iyengar, S. (1989). How citizens think about national issues: A matter of responsibility. *American Journal of Political Science, 33* (4), 878(23).

Jensen, G., & Brownfield, D. (1986). Gender, lifestyles, and victimization: Beyond routine activity. *Violence and Victims,* 1 (2), 85-99.

Jockin, V., Arvey, R., McGue, M. (2001). Perceived victimization moderates self-reports of workplace aggression and conflict. *Journal of Applied Psychology, 86* (6), 1262(8).

Kasper, J., Hoge, S., Feucht-Haviar, T., Cortina, J., & Cohen, B. (1997). Prospective study of patients' refusal of antipsychotic medication under a physician discretion review procedure. *American Journal of Psychiatry, 154* (4), 483-489.

Kennedy, L., & Baron, S. (1993). Routine activities and a subculture of violence: A study of violence on the street. *Journal of Research in Crime and Delinquency,* 30 (1), 88(25).

Kennedy, L., & Forde, D. (1990). Routine activities and crime: An analysis of victimization in Canada. *Criminology,* 28 (1), 137-152.

Kennedy, L., & Silverman, R. (1990). The elderly victim of homicide: An application of the routine activities approach. *Sociological Quarterly, 31* (2), 308(12).

Kline, J., & Sussman, L. (2000). An executive guide to workplace depression. *The Academy of Management Executive, 14* (3), 103.

Labig, C. (1995). *Preventing violence in the workplace.* New York: Amacom.

Laden, V., & Schwartz, G. (2000). Psychiatric disabilities, the americans with disabilities act, and the new workplace violence account. *Berkeley Journal of Employment and Labor Law Summer, 21* (1), 246.

LaMar, W. J., Gerberich, S. G., Lohman, W. H., & Zaidman, B. (1998). Work-related physical assault. *Journal of Occupational and Environmental Medicine, 40* (4), 317(8).

Laschinger, H., Finegan, J., & Shamian, J. (2001). Promoting nurses' health: Effect of empowerment on job strain and work satisfaction. *Nursing Economics, 19* (2), 42.

Lasley, J. (1989). Drinking routines/lifestyles and predatory victimization: A causal analysis. *Justice Quarterly, 6* (4), 529-542.

Lauritsen, J., Sampson, R., & Laub, J. (1991). The link between offending and victimization among adolescents. *Criminology, 29* (2), 265-291.

Lester, M., & Maccone, M. (2001). Prevent violence in the workplace: The work environment must be physically secure with communication and evacuation plans in place. *New Jersey Law Journal, 166* (6), S-1(4).

Lewis-Beck, M. S. (1980). *Applied regression: An introduction.* Newbury Park, CA: Sage Publications, Inc.

Lichtenstein, R., Netemeyer, R., & Burton, S. (1995). Assessing the domain specificity of deal proneness: A field study. *Journal of Consumer Research, 22* (3), 314(13).

Lincoln, K. (2000). Social support, negative social interactions, and psychological well-being. *Social Service Review, 74* (2), 231.

Lindqvist, P., & Allebeck, P. (1990). Schizophrenia and crime: A longitudinal follow-up of 644 schizophrenics in stockholm. *British Journal of Psychiatry, 157,* 345-350.

Link, B., Andrews, H., & Cullen, F. (1992). The violent and illegal behavior of mental patients reconsidered. *American Sociological Review, 57,* 275-292.

Link, B., Monahan, J., Stueve, A., & Cullen, F. (1999). Real in their consequences: A sociological approach to understanding the association between psychotic symptoms and violence. *American Sociological Review, 64* (2), 316(1).

Lynch, J. (1987). Routine activity and victimization at work. *Journal of Quantitative Criminology, 3* (4), 283-300.

Madriz, E. (1996). The perception of risk in the workplace: A test of routine activity theory. *Journal of Criminal Justice, 24* (5), 407(12).

Martell, D., & Dietz, P. (1992). Mentally disordered offenders who push or attempt to push victims onto subway tracks in new york city. *Archives of General Psychiatry, 49,* 472-475.

Marzuk, P. (1996). Violence, crime, and mental illness: How strong a link? *Archives of General Psychiatry 53,* 481-486.

Massey, J., Krohn, M., & Bonati, L. (1989). Property crime and the routine activities of individuals. *Journal of Research in Crime and Delinquency, 26* (4), 378-400.

Maxfield, M. (1987). Household composition, routine activity, and victimization: A comparative analysis. *Journal of Quantitative Criminology, 3* (4), 301-320.

Maxwell, J. (1996). *Qualitative research design: An interactive approach.* Thousand Oaks, CA: Sage Publications, Inc.

McElrath, K., & Chitwood, D. (1997). Crime victimization among injection drug users. *Journal of Drug Issues, 27* (4), 771(13).

McKoy, Y., & Smith, M. (2001). Legal considerations of workplace violence in healthcare environments. *Nursing Forum, 36* (1), 5.

Menard, S. (1995). *Applied logistic regression analysis.* Thousand Oaks, CA: Sage Publications, Inc.

Mertler, C., & Vannatta, R. (2001). Advanced and multivariate statistical methods: Practical application and interpretation. Los Angeles, CA: Pyrczak Publishing.

Messner, S., & Blau, J. (1987). Routine leisure activities and rates of crime: A macro-level analysis. *Social Forces, 65,* 1035-1052.

Messner, S., & Tardiff, K. (1985). The social ecology of urban homicide: An application of the routine activities approach. *Criminology, 23* (2), 241-267.

Miethe, T., & Meier, R. (1990). Opportunity, choice, and criminal victimization: A test of a theoretical model. *Journal of Research in Crime and Delinquency, 27* (3), 243-266.

Miethe, T., Stafford, M., & Long, J. (1987). Social differentiation in criminal victimization: A test of routine activities/lifestyle theories. *American Sociological Review,* 52, 184-194.

Miethe, T., Stafford, M., & Sloane, D. (1990). Lifestyle changes and risks of criminal victimization. *Journal of Quantitative Criminology, 6* (4), 357-376.

Modestin, J., & Ammann, R. (1996). Mental disorder and criminality: Male schizophrenia. *Schizophrenia Bulletin, 22* (1), 69-82.

Moffatt, G. (1998). Subjective fear: Preventing workplace homicide. *HR Focus, 75* (8), 11(2).

Monahan, J. (1992). Mental disorder and violent behavior. *American Psychologist, 47* (4), 511-521.

Monahan, J., & Arnold, J. (1996). Violence by people with mental illness: A consensus statement by advocates and researchers. *Psychiatric Rehabilitation Journal, 19* (4), 67(4).

National Institute for Occupational Safety and Health (1993a). *NIOSH urges immediate action to prevent workplace homicide* (DHHS Publication No. 94-101). Cincinnati, OH: Author.

National Institute for Occupational Safety and Health (1993b). *Preventing homicide in the workplace* (DHHS Publication No. 93-109). Cincinnati, OH: Author.

National Institute for Occupational Safety and Health (1996). *Violence in the workplace: Risk factors and prevention strategies* (DHHS Publication No. 96-100). Cincinnati, OH: Author.

Nigro, L., & Waugh, W. (1996). Violence in the American workplace: Challenges to the public employer. *Public Administration Review, 56* (4), 326-333.

Norstrom, T. (2000). Outlet density and criminal violence in norway, 1960-1995. *Journal of Studies on Alcohol, 61* (6), 907.

O'Loughlin, J., Flint, C., & Anselin, L. (1994). The geography of the nazi vote: Context, confession, and class in the reichstag election of 1930. *The Annals of the Association of American geographers, 84* (3), 351(30).

Osgood, D., Wilson, J., O'Malley, P., Bachman, J., & Johnston, L. (1996). Routine activities and individual deviant behavior. *American Sociological Review, 61* (4), 635-655.

Parker, R., & Toth, A. (1990). Family, intimacy, and homicide: A macro-social approach. *Violence and Victims, 5* (3), 195-210.

Peek-Asa, C., Schaffer, K. B., Kraus, J. F., & Howard, J. (1998). Surveillance of non-fatal workplace assault injuries, using police and employers' reports. *Journal of Occupational and Environmental Medicine, 40* (8), 707(7).

Pindyck, R. S., & Rubinfeld, D. L. (1981). *Econometric models and economic forecasts* (2$^{nd}$ ed.). New York: McGraw-Hill.

Rabkin, J. (1979). Criminal behavior of discharged mental patients: A critical appraisal of the research. *Psychological Bulletin, 86* (1), 1-27.

Racette, K. (2001). Violence in the workplace. *Radiologic Technology, 72* (4), 329.

Rasanen, P., Tiihonen, J., Isohanni, M., Rantakallio, P., Lehtonen, J., & Moring, J. (1998). Schizophrenia, alcohol abuse, and violent behavior: A 26-year follow-up study of an unselected birth cohort. *Schizophrenia Bulletin, 24* (3), 437-441.

Rodgers, K., & Roberts, G. (1995). Women's non-spousal multiple victimization: A test of the routine activities theory. *Canadian Journal of Criminology*, July 1995, 363-391.

Roncek, D., & Maier, P. (1991). Bars, blocks, and crimes revisited: Linking the theory of routine activities to the empiricism of hot spots. *Criminology, 29* (4), 725-753.

Rotton, J., & Cohn, E. (2000). Weather, disorderly conduct, and assaults: From social contact to social avoidance. *Environment and Behavior, 32* (5), 651(23).

Rotton, J., & Cohn, E. (2000a). Violence is a curvilinear function of temperature in dallas: A replication. *Journal of Personality and Social Psychology, 78* (6), 1074.

Rountree, P., & Land, K. (1996). Burglary victimization, perceptions of crime risk, and routine activities: A multilevel analysis across seattle neighborhoods and census tracts. *Journal of Research in Crime and Delinquency, 33* (2), 147(34).

Rountree, P., Land, K., & Miethe, T. (1994). Macro-micro integration in the study of victimization: A hierarchical logistic model analysis across seattle neighborhoods. *Criminology, 32* (3), 387-414.

Rubin, H., & Rubin, I. (1995). *Qualitative interviewing: The art of hearing data.* Thousand Oaks, CA: Sage Publications, Inc.

Sampson, R., & Lauritsen, J. (1990). Deviant lifestyles, proximity to crime, and the offender-victim link in personal violence. *Journal of Research in Crime and Delinquency, 27* (2), 110-139.

Sampson, R., & Wooldredge, J. (1987). Linking the micro- and macro-level dimensions of lifestyle—routine activity and opportunity models of predatory victimization. *Journal of Quantitative Criminology, 3* (4), 371-393.

Satel, S., & Jaffe, D. (1998). Violent fantasies. *National Review, 50* (13), p. 36(2).

Schroeder, L., Sjoquist, D., & Stephan, P. (1986). *Understanding regression analysis: An introductory guide.* Newbury Park: Sage Publications, Inc.

Schwartz, M., & Pitts, V. (1995). Exploring a feminist routine activities approach to explaining sexual assault. *Justice Quarterly, 12* (1), 9-31.

Sherman, L., Gartin, P., & Buerger, M. (1989). Hot spots of predatory crime: Routine activities and the criminology of place. *Criminology, 27* (1), 27-55.

Shore, D., Filson, C., & Rae, D. (1990). Violent crime arrest rates of white house case subjects and matched control subjects. *American Journal of Psychiatry, 147* (6), 746-750.

Smith, L. (1989). Medication refusal and the rehospitalized mentally ill inmate. *Hospital and Community Psychiatry, 40* (5), 491-496.

Smith, W., Frazee, S., & Davison, E. (2000). Furthering the integration of routine activity and social disorganization theories: Small units of analysis and the study of street robbery as a diffusion process. *Criminology, 38* (2), 489(35).

Sosowsky, L. (1980). Explaining increased arrest rate among mental patients: A cautionary note. *American Journal of Psychiatry, 137* (12), 1602-1605.

Southerland, M., Collins, P., & Scarborough, K. (1997). *Workplace violence: A continuum from threat to death.* Cincinnati, OH: Anderson Publishing Company.

Steadman, H., Mulvey, E., Monahan, J., Robbins, P., Appelbaum, P., Grisso, T., Roth, L., & Silver, E. (1998). Violence by people discharged from acute psychiatric inpatient facilities and by others in the same neighborhoods. *Archives of General Psychiatry, 55*, 393-401.

Steinert, T. (2001). Reducing violence in severe mental illness: Community care does not do well. *British Medical Journal, 323* (7321), 1080(2).

Stitt, G., Giacopassi, D., & Vandiver, M. (2000). A minor concern? Underage casino gambling and the law. *The Social Science Journal, 37* (3), 361-73.

Sullivan, C., & Yuan, C. (1995). Workplace assaults on minority health and mental health care workers in Los Angeles. *The American Journal of Public Health, 85* (7), 1011(4).

Sutton, M. (1995). Supply by theft: Does the market for second-hand goods play a role in keeping crime figures high? *British Journal of Criminology, 35*_(3), 400-416.

Swanson, J., Estroff, S., Swartz, M., Borum, R., Lachicotte, W., Zimmer, C., & Wagner, R. (1997). Violence and severe mental disorder in clinical and community populations: The effects of psychotic symptoms, comorbidity, and lack of treatment. *Psychiatry, 60*, 1-22.

Swanson, J., Holzer, C., Ganju, V., Jono, R. (1990). Violence and psychiatric disorder in the community: Evidence from the epidemiologic catchment area surveys. *Hospital and Community Psychiatry, 41* (7), 761-770.

Swartz, M., Swanson, J., Hiday, V., Borum, R., Wagner, R., & Burns, B. (1998). Violence and severe mental illness: The effects of substance abuse and nonadherence to medication. *American Journal of Psychiatry, 155* (2), 226-231.

Taylor, P. (1985). Motives for offending among violent and psychotic men. *British Journal of Psychiatry, 147*, 491-498.

Taylor, P., Leese, M., Williams, D., Butwell, M., Daly, R., & Larkin, E. (1998). Mental disorder and violence: A special (high security) hospital study. *British Journal of Psychiatry, 172*, 218-226.

Terpin, D. (1995). Workplace violence: A growing epidemic. *Safety and Health,152* (4), 252.

Tewksbury, R., & Ehrhardt-Mustaine, E. (2001). Lifestyle factors associated with sexual assault of men: A routine activity theory analysis. *Journal of Men's Studies, 9* (2), 153-182.

Tremblay, M., & Tremblay, P. (1998). Social structure, interaction opportunities, and the direction of violent offenses. *Journal of Research in Crime and Delinquency, 35* (3), 295-315.

Warchol, G. (1998). *Workplace Violence, 1992-1996* (NCJ Publication No. 168634). Washington, D.C.: Bureau of Justice Statistics.

Warshaw, L. J., & Messite, J. (1996). Workplace violence: Preventive and interventive strategies. *Journal of Occupational and Environmental Medicine, 38* (10), 993(14).

Wessely, S., Castle, D., Douglas, A., & Taylor, P. (1994). The criminal careers of incident cases of schizophrenia. *Psychological Medicine, 24,* 483-502.

Wittebrood, K., & Nieuwbeerta, P. (2000). Criminal victimization during one's life course: The effects of previous victimization and patterns of routine activities. *Journal of Research on Crime and Delinquency, 37* (1), 91-122.

Wooldredge, J. (1998). Inmate lifestyles and opportunities for victimization. *Journal of Research in Crime and Delinquency, 35* (4), 480(23).

Wooldredge, J., Cullen, F., & Latessa, E. (1992). Victimization in the workplace. A test of routine activities theory. *Justice Quarterly, 9* (2), 325-335.

# Index

Allebeck, 3, 48, 49, 147
Ammann, 48, 52, 65, 86, 111, 123, 125, 149
Anderson, 2, 44, 56, 58, 139, 154
Andrews, 3, 147
Anselin, 5, 150
Appelbaum, 3, 48, 58, 139, 154
Arango, 48, 52, 65, 86, 111, 123, 125, 139
Arnold, 3, 48, 53, 54, 58, 84, 85, 93, 124, 138, 150
Arseneault, 3, 48, 139
Arvey, 47, 145
Asdigian, 38, 143
Babbie, 73, 76, 78, 79, 139
Bachman, 6, 94, 139, 150
Barba, 48, 139
Baron, 3, 14, 15, 36, 37, 38, 40, 47, 48, 58, 84, 124, 140, 145
Bartels, 48, 51, 86, 93, 124, 125, 140
Bennett, 13, 15, 27, 140
Benson, 77, 143
Blau, 14, 149
Block, 2, 43, 140
Bonati, 5, 148
Borum, 4, 155
Bower, 53, 84, 85, 93, 138, 140
Brennan, 3, 144
Brownfield, 13, 37, 38, 145
Bryant, 5, 18, 20, 40, 60, 74, 140
Buerger, 14, 153
Burns, 4, 155
Burton, 147
Butwell, 49, 155
Calabrese, 47, 140
Cantor, 7, 13, 23, 27, 30, 141
Cao, 14, 38, 140
Capozzoli, 3, 44, 45, 47, 48, 57, 58, 84, 121, 124, 136, 141
Carroll, 44, 45, 87, 141

Caspi, 3, 139
Castle, 49, 156
Chamlin, 14, 38, 141
Chitwood, 14, 33, 148
Cochran, 14, 38, 141
Cohen, 4, 5, 7, 8, 9, 10, 11, 12, 13, 15, 18, 23, 27, 29, 30, 38, 40, 48, 63, 141, 143, 145
Cohn, 14, 152
Collins, 1, 7, 13, 16, 22, 24, 141, 154
Cortina, 48, 145
Cox, 13, 97, 98, 99, 102, 103, 104, 106, 107, 108, 109, 141
Creswell, 64, 142
Cullen, 3, 5, 147, 156
Daly, 49, 155
Davison, 14, 153
DeCoster, 4, 13, 22, 25, 142
Dietz, 48, 51, 85, 86, 93, 148
Domain-Specific, 3, 21
Douglas, 49, 156
Drake, 48, 140
Ehrhardt-Mustaine, 4, 13, 14, 17, 18, 22, 24, 31, 32, 142, 156
Engberg, 3, 144
Eronen, 3, 48, 49, 142
Estes, 4, 142
Estroff, 4, 155
Felson, 2, 4, 5, 7, 8, 9, 10, 11, 12, 13, 18, 29, 38, 40, 43, 63, 140, 141, 142, 143
Feucht-Haviar, 48, 145
Filson, 3, 153
Finch, 4, 143
Finegan, 47, 146
Finkelhor, 38, 143
Flint, 5, 150
Forde, 14, 30, 35, 37, 38, 39, 145
Fowler, 76, 143
Frazee, 14, 153

Freeman, 48, 140
Ganju, 4, 155
Garofalo, 8, 13, 22, 143, 144
Gartin, 14, 153
George, 13, 22, 143
Gerberich, 46, 146
Giacopassi, 13, 22, 154
Gonzalez-Salvador, 48, 139
Gottfredson, 8, 144
Grisso, 4, 154
Guardianship, 5, 23, 28, 85, 114,
    128
Harris, 77, 143
Hashemi, 56, 144
Hawley, 8, 9, 144
Hiday, 4, 155
Hindelang, 8, 13, 29, 30, 144
Hlebovy, 47, 144
Hoag-Apel, 44, 87, 144
Hodgins, 3, 48, 49, 144
Hoge, 48, 145
Holzer, 4, 155
Howard, 3, 151
Isohanni, 49, 151
Iyengar, 4, 145
Jaffe, 55, 153
Jensen, 13, 37, 38, 145
Jockin, 47, 145
Johnston, 6, 150
Jono, 4, 155
Kasper, 48, 51, 86, 93, 145
Kennedy, 13, 14, 15, 30, 32, 33,
    35, 36, 37, 38, 39, 40, 145
Kline, 47, 146
Kluegel, 13, 15, 141
Kraus, 2, 151
Krohn, 5, 148
Labig, 3, 45, 47, 48, 58, 84, 124,
    146
Lachicotte, 4, 155
Laden, 1, 3, 7, 48, 58, 146
LaMar, 46, 56, 66, 67, 68, 113,
    115, 116, 123, 126, 127, 128,
    131, 132, 146
Land, 14, 15, 141, 152

Langan, 13, 141
Larkin, 49, 155
Laschinger, 47, 146
Lasley, 14, 37, 146
Latessa, 5, 156
Laub, 13, 22, 143, 146
Lauritsen, 14, 37, 60, 146, 152
Leese, 49, 155
Lehtonen, 49, 151
Lester, 44, 45, 58, 146
Lewis-Beck, 91, 92, 93, 94, 147
Lichtenstein, 5, 147
Lincoln, 5, 147
Lindqvist, 3, 48, 49, 147
Link, 3, 48, 49, 52, 65, 86, 111,
    123, 125, 147
Logistic Regression, 5, 91, 95, 96,
    97, 98, 102, 103, 107, 109,
    131, 148
Lohman, 46, 146
Long, 6, 149
Lynch, 5, 7, 13, 14, 15, 16, 19, 21,
    22, 23, 24, 30, 40, 59, 68, 74,
    75, 117, 118, 126, 132, 147
Maccone, 44, 45, 58, 146
Madriz, 5, 7, 13, 22, 24, 147
Maier, 18, 152
Martell, 48, 51, 86, 93, 148
Marzuk, 48, 53, 148
Massey, 5, 14, 18, 19, 20, 27, 28,
    29, 30, 40, 60, 74, 148
Maume, 14, 38, 140
Maxfield, 9, 13, 22, 148
Maxwell, 76, 148
McElrath, 14, 33, 148
McGue, 47, 145
McKoy, 2, 58, 148
McVey, 3, 44, 45, 47, 48, 57, 58,
    84, 121, 124, 136, 141
Mednick, 3, 144
Meier, 10, 14, 15, 33, 149
Menard, 94, 95, 148
Mental health, 1, 2, 4, 5, 6, 38, 41,
    44, 47, 48, 52, 56, 58, 59, 60,
    63, 64, 65, 68, 69, 70, 71, 73,

74, 75, 76, 77, 81, 83, 86, 89,
    86, 97, 99, 119, 121, 123, 125,
    126, 128, 129, 131, 135, 136,
    137, 138, 154
Mental illness, 3, 6, 41, 47, 48, 50,
    51, 52, 53, 54, 55, 58, 60, 65,
    70, 85, 86, 112, 123, 125, 148,
    150, 154, 155
Mentally ill, 2, 3, 6, 37, 47, 48, 49,
    52, 53, 54, 55, 58, 65, 66, 69,
    71, 72, 84, 85, 93, 94, 111,
    112, 123, 124, 137, 138, 140,
    153
Mertler, 92, 93, 95, 148
Messite, 3, 44, 46, 47, 48, 57, 59,
    66, 67, 68, 84, 87, 88, 89, 113,
    114, 115, 117, 121, 123, 125,
    126, 127, 128, 131, 132, 136,
    156
Messner, 9, 14, 31, 149
Miethe, 6, 10, 14, 15, 17, 18, 20,
    27, 29, 30, 33, 34, 35, 39, 40,
    60, 149, 152
Miller, 5, 18, 20, 40, 60, 74, 140
Modestin, 48, 52, 65, 86, 111,
    123, 125, 149
Moffatt, 45, 149
Moffitt, 3, 139
Monahan, 3, 37, 48, 49, 53, 54,
    58, 84, 85, 93, 124, 138, 139,
    147, 149, 150, 154
Moring, 49, 151
Motivated offenders, 4, 6, 8, 11,
    12, 16, 18, 20, 28, 40, 60
Mueller, 4, 142
Mulvey, 4, 154
National Institute for Occupational
    Safety and Health, 43, 150
Netemeyer, 5, 147
Neuman, 3, 47, 48, 58, 84, 124,
    140
Nieuwbeerta, 15, 16, 156
Nigro, 3, 45, 46, 47, 48, 57, 58,
    66, 67, 68, 84, 113, 115, 116,

121, 123, 125, 126, 127, 128,
    130, 131, 132, 136, 150
Norstrom, 13, 22, 150
O'Loughlin, 5, 150
O'Malley, 6, 150
OLS, 5, 91, 92, 95, 96, 100, 105,
    110
Ordonez, 48, 139
Ormrod, 38, 143
Osgood, 6, 18, 40, 60, 150
Parker, 14, 38, 151
Paternoster, 94, 139
Peek-Asa, 2, 44, 45, 56, 57, 58,
    59, 88, 94, 120, 123, 135, 151
Pindyck, 93, 151
Pitts, 6, 14, 18, 39, 40, 60, 153
Potential Offenders, 5, 84, 111,
    123
Rabkin, 3, 49, 151
Racette, 44, 151
Rae, 3, 153
Rantakallio, 49, 151
Rasanen, 49, 151
Robbins, 3, 139, 154
Roberts, 14, 32, 151
Rodgers, 14, 32, 151
Roncek, 18, 152
Roth, 4, 154
Rotton, 14, 152
Rountree, 14, 38, 152
Routine activities, 2, 3, 4, 5, 6, 7,
    8, 9, 10, 13, 14, 15, 16, 17, 18,
    19, 21, 22, 23, 24, 25, 26, 27,
    28, 29, 30, 31, 32, 33, 34, 35,
    36, 37, 38, 39, 40, 43, 59, 60,
    63, 68, 73, 74, 92, 111, 117,
    118, 122, 123, 132, 133, 134,
    138, 140, 142, 143, 145, 149,
    151, 152, 153, 156, 157
Rubin, 73, 76, 77, 152
Rubinfeld, 93, 151
Sampson, 14, 37, 39, 60, 146, 152,
    153
Satel, 55, 153
Scarborough, 1, 7, 154

Schaffer, 2, 151
Schroeder, 93, 153
Schulsinger, 3, 144
Schwartz, 1, 3, 6, 7, 14, 18, 39, 40, 48, 58, 60, 146, 153
Shamian, 47, 146
Sherman, 14, 15, 18, 40, 153
Shore, 3, 49, 153
Siegel, 13, 22, 143
Silva, 3, 139
Silver, 4, 154
Silverman, 14, 32, 33, 145
Sjoquist, 93, 153
Sloane, 14, 34, 149
Smith, 2, 14, 49, 51, 58, 86, 93, 148, 153
Sosowsky, 3, 49, 154
Southerland, 1, 2, 7, 8, 43, 58, 154
Stafford, 6, 14, 34, 149
Stamper, 2, 44, 56, 58, 139
Steadman, 4, 53, 54, 84, 85, 93, 138, 154
Steinert, 3, 48, 59, 154
Stephan, 153
Stitt, 13, 22, 154
Stueve, 3, 147
Sullivan, 44, 57, 87, 154
Sussman, 47, 146
Sutton, 6, 18, 40, 60, 154
Swanson, 3, 49, 50, 86, 125, 155
Swartz, 4, 49, 51, 86, 93, 155
Tardiff, 9, 14, 31, 149
Target Suitability, 5, 87, 115, 130
Taylor, 3, 49, 51, 52, 65, 86, 93, 111, 123, 125, 139, 155, 156
Terpin, 3, 155
Tewksbury, 13, 14, 17, 18, 22, 24, 142, 156
Thomas, 13, 22, 143

Tiihonen, 3, 49, 142, 151
Toth, 14, 38, 151
Tremblay, 9, 156
Vandiver, 13, 22, 154
Vannatta, 92, 93, 95, 148
Violence in the workplace, 1, 2, 8, 41, 46, 47, 57, 58, 59, 64, 72, 75, 81, 84, 93, 121, 123, 137, 141, 144, 146 151
Wagner, 4, 155
Wallach, 48, 140
Warchol, 1, 2, 3, 43, 44, 45, 56, 58, 89, 94, 120, 123, 135, 156
Warshaw, 3, 44, 46, 47, 48, 57, 59, 66, 67, 68, 84, 87, 88, 89, 113, 114, 115, 117, 121, 123, 125, 126, 127, 128, 131, 132, 136, 156
Waugh, 3, 45, 46, 47, 48, 57, 58, 66, 67, 68, 84, 113, 115, 116, 121, 123, 125, 126, 127, 128, 130, 131, 132, 136, 150
Webster, 56, 144
Wessely, 49, 52, 65, 86, 111, 123, 125, 156
Williams, 49, 155
Wilson, 6, 150
Wittebrood, 15, 16, 156
Wooldredge, 5, 13, 22, 25, 26, 37, 39, 60, 126, 153, 156
Workplace violence, 1, 2, 3, 6, 8, 45, 46, 56, 57, 58, 59, 76, 82, 83, 89, 119, 121, 124, 136, 137, 139, 140, 144, 146, 148, 154, 155, 156
Yuan, 44, 57, 87, 154
Zaidman, 46, 146
Zimmer, 4, 155